Ingrid Noll

Ingrid Noll was born in Shanghai in 1935, but later moved to Bonn and studied German and Art History there. Hailed as 'Germany's Queen of Crime' (*Observer*), Ingrid Noll is the author of three crime novels – *Hell Hath No Fury*, *Head Count* and *The Pharmacist* – which have been translated into more than ten languages and won acclaim worldwide.

INGRID NOLL

THE PHARMACIST

Translated from the German by
IAN MITCHELL

HarperCollins*Publishers*

HarperCollins*Publishers*
77–85 Fulham Palace Road,
Hammersmith, London W6 8JB

This paperback edition 1999

1 3 5 7 9 8 6 4 2

First published in Great Britain by
HarperCollins*Publishers* 1998

First published in Germany with the title
Die Apothekerin
by Diogenes Verlag AG Zürich in 1994

Copyright © 1994 by Diogenes Verlag AG Zürich

Ingrid Noll asserts the moral right to
be identified as the author of this work

ISBN 0 00 649768 3

Set in Meridien and Bodoni

Printed and bound in Great Britain by
Caledonian International Book Manufacturing Ltd, Glasgow

For Gregor

1

Other than the family motto, 'You don't talk about money, you just have it,' and an inexplicable hollow vanity, my mother had inherited nothing from her clan. Towards my father, her attitude was one of submissiveness; in his absence, on the other hand, she could sometimes puff herself up to tyrannosaurus proportions. This became evident to us children only at that time when, for no discernible reason whatsoever, my father renounced all lusts of the flesh to such a degree that he became a vegetarian and tried, with missionary zeal, to convert his family to this cause, too. Nevertheless, out of consideration for our physical development and a certain compassion, he did allow us a little pork and veal sausage, an egg on Sundays or a few crumbs of mince in our Milanese sauce.

Where other housewives would usually brew up a cup of coffee around four in the afternoon, our portly little mother prepared something approaching a carnivore's orgy for herself and for my brother and me. It was the one and only display of conviviality she could ever be accused of, and we took a quite dreadful delight in it.

Every single left-over scrap of meat had to be got out of the way before Father came home – it was like disposing of a body. Nothing, neither bones nor rind, no blobs of fat or even kitchen smells or dirty dishes were to be left to testify to our covert crime. Teeth were cleaned, the waste-bin emptied and the kitchen restored to a state of innocence with a lemon air-freshener.

Yet, deep down, I was a Daddy's girl, and this carnal infidelity caused me great suffering. Had his conversion not come about a good year before the great traumatic experience of my childhood, I would have blamed myself for it.

My father, too, was a great one for pithy maxims where money was concerned. We learned, from an early age, that money is not the root of all evil, nor are the streets paved with it, that it makes the world go round but it doesn't bring happiness. Most often, however, he would mutter, 'Money isn't something you talk about.' He spent it as he saw fit; when my brother was eleven and wanted to learn to play the piano, a concert grand was bought without the batting of an eyelid, and to this day it still dominates my parents' living room, even though, as it turned out, it took a hammering for no more than eight months in all. Yet, against that, Father insisted that I pay for my set square, magic markers, hairgrips and tennis shoes out of my own pocket money. Even my mother had no idea how much her husband earned, but proceeded from the assumption that he was in the top income bracket. Since money was not something you talked about in our house, she occasionally had to couch her demands in coded hints. And yet, when I passed my final school exams and got my *Abitur*, my father presented me with a small car, which was in fact what my brother had been wanting.

I had learnt at an early age that parental love can be bought by achievements. My parents were proud of my good school reports, of my industriousness and of my first successes as a housewife.

There are photos of me doing my bit in the garden, with a dinky little straw hat on my head and a watering can in my hand. My father also snapped me in the rôle of cook, in a large checked apron, delicately decorating sand-pies with toothpaste, and, last but not least, as a nurse. All my dolls and teddy bears are laid out on my cot, their broken limbs swathed in enormous toilet-paper bandages. Some of them are suffering from measles, their faces spotted with red chalk. I can recall only one single occasion when this nurse-syndrome gave rise to an argument between my parents, and that stemmed from my dedicated attempts to apply the kiss of life to a far from recently deceased mole.

In those days, I still imagined myself to be the darling of the family, an industrious, nice little girl, happily dressed in little headscarves. When I started school, too, I fulfilled all expectations; a pupil who showed interest and who later shone particularly in science subjects. When I was still only ten, I collected plants, pressing them and arranging them in a herbarium, which I have to this day. Everything about myself and my possessions had to be neat and tidy and well-ordered, my room was a model of tidiness, my playmates were selected in my own image, my earthworm culture in the cellar was hygienically screened off from the apples stored there.

In secondary school, my achievement-orientated attitude singularly failed to earn the approval of my classmates. My idiosyncrasy of conscientiously underlining important sentences in my textbooks with a ruler and highlighting them with a magic marker became the subject of ridicule, 'swot's yellow fever' they all called it. I tried vainly to make friends. Constant praise from my teachers only made my situation worse.

I was twelve when it happened. During a short break, the teacher left the room, and I too hurried out to go to the toilet, something my nervousness brought on all too often. When I returned and tried to get back into the classroom, the door refused to open. At least a dozen children were pushing against it from the inside; I could hear their muffled whispering and giggling. I wasn't usually one to panic easily, but on that fateful January day I had had a thoroughly miserable morning, and now I could no longer hold back the tears. With all my might, I hurled myself at the chipped grey-painted wooden door which was isolating me from everyone else. The next lesson was due to begin any moment; all I would have needed to do was wait for the bell to ring, and they would all have rushed to their places to sit looking innocent as the teacher made her entry. But I took the situation far too seriously and made a run at the door.

It gave way as if it had never been held shut at all, and I shot into the room like a cannonball. I could feel the pain where the handle had dug hard into my hand, then I crashed down on the green linoleum floor just as the teacher came in. Like will-o'-the-wisps, my foes flitted away to their places.

Naturally, I was cross-questioned by the teacher. I gave nothing away; telling on anyone would never have been forgiven. Soon, peace and quiet was restored, but one boy was missing. 'Axel just staggered out,' my neighbour claimed. The teacher sent someone out to look for him, but they came back empty-handed. Finally, she herself went out into the corridor, called out to him and then, conscientiously carrying out her supervisory duties to the full, even went into the boys' toilets. In the end, somebody suggested Axel had probably run off home because he was afraid I would put the blame on him. Since he was always finding some excuse for playing truant, this seemed quite plausible.

Four hours later, Axel was discovered. As the postmortem showed, I had rammed the door handle into his skull with full force. Unfortunately, he had been peering through the keyhole just at the very moment when the others let the door go without warning. Axel, dazed by a searing pain in his head, had hidden in the map-store, no doubt for fear of being punished. He later died as a result of a massive brain haemorrhage.

There followed a police investigation, of which I can remember hardly anything. When the first, more or less anonymous, notes started landing on my desk, with the word MURDERESS scrawled on the ragged scraps of blue-ruled paper, my parents took me away from that school and put me in another.

At times, I would catch my father gazing steadily at me, with tears and an infinite weariness in his eyes.

So I was removed from that school and stuck in a girls' grammar school run by Ursuline nuns, where I conformed and behaved myself. Whatever you do, just try not to attract attention, was my motto. In fact, there were no signs of hostility towards me; my new school lay in a different part of town, and word of Axel's murder had not got around. I was seen as a rather boring member of the class, and that suited me fine. And that was the way things stayed until I was sixteen and a vague desire stirred in me to find a male counterpart.

The memory of all that still plagues me now, day and night, as I lie here, unable to get away.

You don't get much rest in this hospital where, even as a first-class private patient, you have to share a two-bedded room whether you like it or not. I can't even get on with reading something worthwhile. The constant interruptions by the nursing staff, the endless round of temperature-taking, pill-swallowing (for want of any other kind of pleasures of the flesh!), the waiting for awful meals, the more or less involuntary eavesdropping on other people's visitors, all that constricts the days in a rigid corset. We usually put the light out early. Then, like Scheherazade, I start telling the story of more and more special details of my life; I suppose my room-mate, Frau Hirte, has, by comparison, nothing in the way of intimate secrets to impart. You can't expect an exciting love-life or any real scandal from an ageing spinster. She's here in the Heidelberg Gynaecological Clinic because she's had a hysterectomy. She insists it's only a benign tumour that's playing up a bit. I think it's cancer.

It's a good thing Pavel brought me the photo albums. I often look at myself in them – a really worthwhile alternative to reading. Now and then I even show my neighbour some of the pictures. With her fifty-eight years and her blue-rinsed hair, she is in stark contrast to myself. Almost the only visitor she ever has is an even older woman, who talks of practically nothing but her dog and her own hospital experiences. Whenever Pavel comes to see me, Frau Hirte watches him, not without a certain weary interest; while we chat quietly, she pretends to be asleep, but I'm convinced she's listening in to my visitors, just as I eavesdrop on hers.

My neighbour now knows all about the stigma of being a murderess, with which I was branded at the age of twelve. She listened to that episode with undisguised curiosity.

Probably the reason I'm telling this woman, a complete stranger, about my life is that it's a kind of therapy for me, which, by contrast to sessions on the famous couch, costs nothing. At any rate, I notice that it does help me if I confide in a stranger whom I'll probably never see again, sharing my experiences with a mother confessor in the dim twilight of our hospital room.

11

I would have been quite happy to be on first-name terms, but, as the younger of the two, it was not my place to make the offer. As a first move, I suggested she just call me Hella, but she sent me off with a flea in my ear. What else can you expect from a woman who even addresses her so-called friend as 'Frau Römer'?

'If you were seventeen, Frau Moormann, I might consider it . . .'

That riled me. 'Well, really, you're old enough to be my mother.'

I had obviously touched a raw nerve with that. There was a glint behind her spectacles. But on the whole we get on reasonably well. I find it a bit weird that this woman should be mourning the loss of her womb, and yet she puts up with the pain like a brave little soldier. After all, the organ that has been removed is about as much use at her age as a goitre.

Sometimes, when she goes off to the toilet, I have a root around among her belongings in the drawer of her bedside table or in her locker. From a letter from her health insurance company I've found out such things as her date of birth, marital status (single) and her first name (Rosemarie), but there's nothing in the way of personal letters or photographs. Jewellery and cash, as she told me herself, she has deposited in the hospital safe. It was stupidity, she said, to leave items of any real value lying about the room unattended. Poor she certainly isn't, otherwise she would never have been able to afford the extra premiums for first-class treatment. And besides, her perfume, her nightdresses and her dressing gown are all expensive and in extremely good taste.

Recently I was telling her how, while still just a young thing, I led a double life. In the dark, I couldn't make out her expression, but I was sure she was pulling a sour face.

I kept falling for men who were having an even harder time of it than I was. While my improper escapades never did come to the attention of my teachers or my classmates, I was unable to hide them from my horrified family. Without doubt, I broke my father's heart at that time. His innocent blonde child was hanging about with queer fish and lame ducks who would have been better kept out of his sight. And, to make matters worse, I didn't grow out of this even during adolescence. Just as, when I was small, I would unscrew my dolls' legs in order to patch them up again, so, later on, I would trawl up men who had gone off the straight and narrow and try to restore them. It helped me get over my own problems better if I had the strength to redeem strangers.

In the photos of me as a child, I have a very alert, not to say mischievous look on my face. My brown eyes are taking everything in. Now I try to read what is in them – were they even then sending out messages of that desire to earn love through my own lavishing of care and protection? That extremely feminine urge, which is normally directed towards small children, but can also be sublimated in gardening, cooking and nursing, seemed, in my case, to seek out male victims. In those days, my parents should have let me go baby-sitting, or bought me a horse. Instead, they used to frame my school reports.

At first, I was quite unaware of the magnetic pull that outcasts, the sick and the neurotic exerted on me. Even while I was still at school, I had a boyfriend who was hooked on heroin and looked to me for salvation. In those days, I used to devour chocolate by the pound, sitting through the night talking with my whining sweetheart, and I stole from my parents – money, cigarettes, alcohol. If he hadn't ended up in prison, I'd still be working on his withdrawal to this day. At that time, I was as faithful and loyal as any dog.

The next one was an out-of-work seafarer, and it's no surprise that my catalogue of flotsam includes even the depressive, the chronically sick, the suicide rescued in the nick of time and the ex-convict with a vulture tattooed on his chest.

My professional activities as a pharmacist, too, have enriched my collection. In defiance of all the regulations, I once opened up, to a man racked by pain and in urgent need of medication in the middle of the night, not merely the slot for slipping the prescriptions through, but the shop door itself.

In an attempt to get my own rôle in these tragedies clear in my mind for once and for all, I have repeatedly taken up courses of therapy, but have always broken them off again. Healing those under my own wing took up all my time. And anyway, I didn't need a therapist to tell me that

I, the outwardly upright me, was just drawn to everything that stood beyond the pale of respectable society.

I was troubled by this abyss within myself; sometimes I would dream of being murdered by one of my lovers, of having died without ever having borne a child. Then I would wake up with a sense of worthlessness, for a life without motherhood seemed to me a complete waste. For all my intelligence and all my ability, I have always known full well that the animal side of me was equally important. I was determined to experience, at least once in my lifetime, what it would be like to be at one with creation and to give birth. The sands of time were running. A child meant a great deal to me: a tiny being which you can mould according to your own lights, with which you can carry on just as you please, which you are free to protect and shower with presents to your heart's content. My child would have a part in everything that dictated the course of my life. It would want for nothing, from love to hairgrips. I wanted to be able to see to it that it had an exemplary daddy to look up to, one with a respectable job and a steady income, who came of a good family and was endowed with intelligence. For this purpose, the company I was keeping in those days was totally out of the question.

Frau Hirte was snoring.

2

One Sunday, Dorit, who has been my friend since our young days, came to see me. She can only come if her husband, Gero, looks after the children. Right in the middle of our chat, in tramped the doctor on his rounds. Tactfully, Dorit went out into the corridor. The usual, standard questions: 'How are we today? The varicose veins playing up? Are the stitches hurting?'

'When can I go home?' asked Frau Hirte.

The ward doctor doesn't like taking decisions; she should know him well enough by now. With a glance at the bag of urine hanging from her bed, he said, with some sarcasm, 'So, you'd like us to discharge you complete with a permanent catheter, would you?'

When Dorit was sitting by me once again, I told her how we couldn't stand that Dr Kaiser – for once, Frau Hirte nodded in agreement – not like Dr Johannsen, the senior physician. 'But', I said to Dorit, 'he looks into your eyes for just those two seconds too long, and then you know you could all too easily fall for him.'

My friend laughed and, in her pert, amiable way, drew Frau Hirte into the conversation. 'Hella's right there, don't you think?'

With a grunt, my dried-up neighbour took out her Sunday paper and started reading the business pages.

You can spend days, or for that matter nights, talking about your own family, but most women prefer listening to gossip about affairs. I am assuming that Frau Hirte hasn't very long to live and so won't blow the gaff on me, so I'm happy to grant her a few more exciting, sleepless hours. Most of the time, she has no comment to pass on my tales, although once she did let out a 'You're off your head.' I found that funny; I like to string her along a bit, the old prune. So I told her all about Levin, sparing no details.

*   *   *

When I became friendly with him, I believed at first that my redeemer phase was over. Here, I had a perfectly normal boyfriend, admittedly a few years younger than me and still a student, but for all that, it seemed, a model of middle-class respectability. In my innermost heart, my thoughts turned to marriage, to children, but I would never have come out into the open with such plans. With a young man, you have to give him time.

Levin hadn't always had things easy, but that didn't make him turn straight to crime; he neither resorted to drugs or drink nor to sleeping around. The fact that, immediately after the sudden death of his father, his mother had gone off to Vienna with another man hurt him deeply. Not far from Heidelberg, hardly half an hour away from us, lived a hardy, cantankerous old grandfather, who used his only grandson principally for running his errands, trimming his hedges and chauffeuring him around. Significantly, it was when I was shopping around for a second-hand car that I met Levin.

As possessions, cars are in my book about on a par with washing machines. All that interests me, apart from the price and the number of kilometres on the clock, is the colour – and that has to be nothing conspicuous.

As I was having a look round the dealer's forecourt, this beanpole of a young man was sauntering about, eyeing up the offers on the cards behind the windscreens. I paid no attention and went to look for a salesman to get some information.

'That would be something for you,' said the young man, pointing to a convertible.

I shook my head.

'Have you ever driven in an open-top?' he asked. 'And let the wind blow about your pretty face?'

Taken aback, I stared at him.

'What did they offer you for your old car?' he asked.

'Two thousand,' I said, and could have kicked myself.

When we went into the saleroom together, I let him do the talking. I'm afraid I feel uncomfortable when it comes to arguing about prices. Levin haggled like a horse-trader.

While I was impressed by the result of his efforts, I really didn't want such a flashy car.

Quite against my will, I ended up sitting in the passenger seat on a test drive, while Levin drove and the salesman in the back seat yelled into my ear about the car's merits.

'Why do you wear your hair so short?' asked Levin. 'Fair hair like yours would look terrific, blowing in the wind . . .'

'Look, buy the convertible yourself, since you fancy it so much. And let your own fair hair flutter in the breeze . . .'

'When you're a student, all you can do is dream of that kind of thing.'

So that explained the shabby bomber jacket from the second-hand shop. Poor lad.

Two hours later, the garish red convertible was parked outside my flat, and I had signed a hire-purchase agreement.

In the days that followed, I was plagued by the suspicion that Levin had been secretly working for the car dealer – when it comes to horse-trading, people get up to all sorts of tricks. But I was wrong.

One Sunday morning, this beanpole descended on me. 'A lovely day like this . . .' he started off.

I explained I was busy working at my doctoral thesis, which was why I was doing only half-days in the chemist's shop, and actually I needed to spend the weekend writing if I was to get the thing finished at last.

Levin took the wheel. He had brought me a pair of sunglasses as a present, the kind of thing you pick up at the flea market which, he said, made me look like some sixties film star. People can say what they like about me, that I've a heart of gold and I'm fun to be with, but compliments about my outward appearance are something I take with a pinch of salt.

As it turned out, however, Levin was no mere charmer. He had that positive quality of childlike enthusiasm. 'I've never seen such a beautiful garden!' he exclaimed when, after our drive, he had a good look round my flat. And yet my balcony was no different from a thousand others stuck on to two-bedroomed flats in modern blocks. All the same, I'm very keen on flowers; yellow, red and orange nasturtiums tumbled in my window-boxes, while roses, geraniums and even lilies blossomed in tubs, and the metal spars of the balcony itself were delicately entwined with white sweet peas.

To prolong his visit a little more, I offered to sew on a button that had been torn off.

No thanks, he could do that himself. 'It would be a poor show for a dentist if he wasn't clever with his fingers.'

Surprised, I asked why he was studying dentistry; it didn't seem to be quite him.

'For the same reason you're a pharmacist,' Levin said. 'To make lots of money.' I looked at him, curious; so that's what he thought of me?

On our next trip, we got on first-name terms, but we didn't get as far as sweet nothings. On his third visit, he appeared with a young cat in his arms, which he presented to me, beaming all over his face. I have to admit, there's hardly anything I find more delightful than kittens. I had often been offered one, but I had always rejected them out of a sense of responsibility. I was out all day, I often had night duty or wanted to go off on trips – who would look after the animal then? Levin turned a deaf ear to my misgivings. 'He's a tom. What name are you going to give him?'

I remembered my grandfather's cat which I had so loved as a child, and said, 'Tinker.'

'No, I don't like that,' declared Levin. 'We'll call him Tamerlane.'

So now I had a convertible and a cat, neither of which I had chosen for myself. And sooner rather than later I also had a young man in my bed.

I kept on asking myself whether all that really interested Levin was driving around with the top down. In our relationship, the car played an erotically stimulating rôle, for him at any rate. For me, though, he was the first male friend with whom I could have a laugh and feel young again. Naturally, I never asked whether Levin had already had many women, but it struck me as unlikely. We slept together fairly regularly, but he devoted much more time to conversation. Usually I was the one who made the first move towards any hour of intimacy – although I suppose ten minutes would be nearer the mark.

Sometimes we would drive as far as Frankfurt to go to the cinema. It seemed to me an awful waste of time, especially when the same film was showing here in Heidelberg. Still, it was fun roaring around with someone in a perpetual state of euphoria.

To tell the truth, those were great times. I had promised myself I would neither feed Levin nor water him, neither rock him to sleep nor iron his shirts or so much as do his typing for him. But then he was always busying himself with my car – he put in two loudspeakers and a nearly-new radio – he would take the rubbish downstairs when he was leaving or bring the cat fish scraps from the Nordsee snack bar he frequented. I couldn't be so hard-hearted as to refuse to fry up steak and onions for the poor skinny lad; they so seldom served decent meat in the students' refectory. Obligingly, I would clean the bathtub and buy socks and underpants, so that there would be something clean for him to put on after his herbal bath. I was getting hardly any work done on my dissertation now. Levin tried to keep me from it, saying he thought a doctorate was quite unnecessary for a pharmacist. I explained that, at the chemist's, I was working as little more than a sales assistant (with computer competence), but with an authentic qualification behind me I'd have the chance of getting a job in industry or in research.

'Where is the best money to be earned?'

'Probably in industry, or obviously if I had my own chemist's shop. What I'd like most of all would be an academic post, preferably something in the field of toxicology.' I was careful not to give him an inkling of what I really wanted more than anything.

Every three weeks, I had night duty; then Levin liked to come in and see me and have me explain what I had to do. 'It's nothing very exciting, really,' I said. 'In my grandfather's chemist's shop, they still used to make up a lot of prescriptions according to the doctor's directions,

19

but I'm afraid I'm only allowed to do that for one or two dermatologists now.'

Sadly, I had inherited nothing other than a few bottles and mortars from my grandfather's equipment, since his shop had been sold. Levin wanted to see my legacy; one thing that still rankles to this day is the fact that I wasn't left Grandfather's collection of walking sticks. In his time, men didn't go about with briefcases or executive cases, but had their hands free for walking sticks or umbrellas. Nowadays, collectors are always on the hunt for valuable antique pieces, the sort of thing my grandfather used to talk his customers into parting with for a few coppers. He owned one doctor's walking stick with a coiled snake in carved ivory, a rosewood and enamel opera cane, ebony and horn sticks with silver, bronze, tortoiseshell and mother-of-pearl knobs. I can remember dragons' and lions' heads which held a gruesome fascination for me as a child, as well as a short dagger-stick and a sword-stick. My father sold the lot.

I took the beautiful brown glass bottles with the handwritten labels down from the hat shelf in my wardrobe.

'Would you give me one of those as a present?' he begged. 'I'd like to keep my aftershave in it.'

It goes without saying that he chose my favourite little bottle, the smallest and finest of them all. On the faded label, in violet ink, the word POISON was still legible. Levin's interest was roused. With an effort, he tugged out the cut-glass stopper and shook the contents on to a silk sofa cushion. Tiny glass tubes with the diameter of a nail and between two and four centimetres in length slid out. Levin read 'Apomorphine Hydrochlor., Special Formula No. 5557, Physostygmine Salicyl. gr. 1/600, Poisons List Great Britain, Schedule 1,' and so on. He looked at me, inquiringly. 'Poison?'

'Obviously,' I said. 'Nothing out of the ordinary, for a chemist.'

With great care, Levin opened one of these miniature doll's tubes, withdrew the cotton wool and took out one of the tablets. Even I was amazed at how tiny it was, smaller than the pupil of an eye.

Levin said he found it an interesting fact that in totalitarian states politicians or people entrusted with secrets went about with a poison capsule hidden in a hollow tooth, so as to be able, in an emergency, to evade torture by committing suicide. 'But I had no idea how dainty poison can look . . .'

I took the tubes from him, rinsed the flacon with soapy boiling water and handed it back to him.

Later on, he gave me a ticking-off for having stored such dangerous stuff for years in my wardrobe. I had had more than a few suicide candidates spending the night here in the past; it was a good thing that these days were over. I looked for a new hiding place for my poison, tipped the lavender from a scented cushion into the dustbin, pushed the tiny tubes in instead and fastened the cushion with a safety pin into the inside of a long woollen skirt that I seldom wore.

Dorit, my friend from my student days, is kept pretty busy by two small children. Unfortunately, I see her only very seldom, like when she's out of Valium again. Then she makes the most of the chance to give me a good talking-to. We were sitting in our favourite café when I had to listen to her telling me yet again that I shouldn't bury myself in my work, otherwise I'd never manage to get myself a husband and a family.

'Listen, Dorit, at the moment I can hardly get any work done at all. I've got a new boyfriend . . .'

'Really? I hope it's not another of these dead losses!'

I promised to introduce him to her.

Levin was twenty-seven, but unfortunately gave the impression of being much younger. He still had a schoolboy's gangling figure, the appetite of a fourteen-year-old and the capacity for enthusiasm of a school beginner. He was good-looking, or so I thought, but not to the extent where all women would throw themselves at him, for his rosy childish features, in which the nose seemed too large, were slightly lopsided. His conscientious application to his studies, his

21

ambition of completing them as soon as possible, did not altogether match his youthful qualities.

As was only to be expected, Dorit was dissatisfied.

'I have to grant you, he is something of an improvement,' she said, 'but he won't marry you. With all *your* experience in love affairs, you must be able to see that for yourself.'

'And why not?'

'Oh, heavens, we've both seen it before. He's looking for a mummy to bring him cough-sweets from the chemist's shop and lend him her car. There will come a time when you'll be on your way home from work, tired out, and you'll spot him sitting down by the River Neckar, holding hands with some twenty-year-old.'

Dorit meant well, and she wasn't altogether wrong; even I had such visions of horror from time to time. But who is going to kick out the man she loves, just out of pure common sense? And anyway, the age difference between us was not excessive. What are eight years these days, when women often marry men twenty years their junior? In any case, I looked younger than my age. Dorit even used to claim that I was one of those blonde women who look as good at fifty-five as they did at twenty-five, but that's a prophecy that has still to be fulfilled. (What a good thing it was that I had been wearing contact lenses for two years and Levin had never seen me in my large glasses.) Of course, there was something else which stood between us, but I couldn't quite put a name to it. I didn't take his passion for cars all that seriously, but occasionally a tendency to superficiality did strike me as disagreeable. Even his capacity for enthusiasm didn't go very far, since as a rule it was directed merely at external things.

Nevertheless, whenever I drove out with Levin on a sunny Sunday for a meal in Alsace, life, it seemed to me, was just perfect.

One afternoon, as we were sitting on the sofa eating home-baked cherry tart, Dorit called by with her children – no doubt to take a good look at our idyll for herself. Immediately, an argument broke out between the children as to who was to get to stroke the cat.

'I've never seen such sweet children,' enthused Levin, even though Franz had just pulled out a tuft of his sister's hair and Tamerlane had fled spitting to take refuge on top of the cupboard.

Dorit was never known for her shyness. With her voice like a rusty door hinge, she came straight out and inquired of my young boyfriend, 'How many children do you want to have in the end?'

I went so red that I had to turn my attention to the cat; I just couldn't look at Levin.

Without turning a hair, he replied, 'Two, probably.'

I could have thrown my arms round his neck and kissed him, but then who said a word about me being the projected mother of these two children?

When Levin took the coffee pot out to the kitchen, Dorit twinkled her eyes at me, and I gestured to her that I could happily strangle her.

Nevertheless, I let her into the secret – since I would have had to tell her sooner or later anyway – that I would shortly be working full-time in the chemist's, at first as replacement for a colleague going off on maternity leave, and so, as long as that went on, my dissertation would have to be put on hold. But I didn't say a word to her about having started typing up Levin's doctoral thesis for him. That was precisely what should not have happened, but when he had asked me to show him how my computer worked, he acted pretty stupid, to put it mildly. Levin, the expert all-round handyman, had never managed anything more advanced on a PC than children's games.

Yet I have to admit that I was happy. Although the subject matter was alien to me, his work appeared to be more straightforward than mine. I pored over reference books and got to know all about completely new aspects of the human jaw. Even now, after such a long time, I could still give a short talk on, say, 'Silicon impression materials and their application in the mouth'.

It was no doubt Father's vegetarianism that made me into a great fan of meat dishes, even though I have since learned that too much of that can be bad for you. A hundred grams per person, that's all I buy; nevertheless, for a hungry young man I was prepared to make an exception. And then, whenever we got stuck into a gigantic T-bone steak together, we would be in high spirits.

One day, Levin brought me a carving knife and a serving fork in monogrammed family silver. Touched, I examined the delicate Greek interlace pattern, the entwined initials and the small traces of everyday use which three generations had left on the blade of the knife.

'Gorgeous,' I said. 'I can hardly imagine your grandfather being willing to part with it.'

'Well, not directly,' said Levin, sharpening the knife on a steel; his grandfather didn't need things like that any more, since he persisted with an ill-fitting set of dentures – out of meanness, he said – and all his meat dishes had to be cooked through till they were as soft as butter.

'I don't think that's right,' I said firmly. 'I can't take any pleasure in stolen goods. Take them straight back to him.'

Levin had a good laugh at that. He would inherit the stuff anyway; surely we weren't going to let such beautiful silver just go to waste, were we?

I gave in, putting the whole thing out of my mind as a belated schoolboy prank, and quickly became accustomed to these pieces of cutlery which, as time passed, became more numerous.

My friend Dorit would always scoff whenever I preached to her on the vainity of all material values. Dorit frankly admitted that she liked buying expensive things. She accused me of insincerity. But I think it would be better described as understatement: I just hate swank. All the same, I do sometimes feel tempted to blow a thousand marks on the odd small item – like a Japanese netsuke figurine, for example, or a delicate Art Nouveau ring in pearls and enamel, or maybe an absolutely exquisite handbag. Which was why I couldn't really bring myself to make any serious objections when Levin brought me pieces of his grandmother's jewellery. They were modest items, finely worked, but always pure gold. After all, I was doing a lot for him, spending money on him and trying to share his interests. Silver cutlery and gold knick-knacks were tokens of his love, that's the way you had to look at it. There was still the matter of a child to be settled.

Most of my classmates had already started a family or were getting on in a career. We were all a bit sorry for Vera, the first one to have to get married right after the finals. There she had been, still only twenty, with no training whatsoever, but with an untimely baby. At that age, we had our minds on other things, went on trips to America or started out on a free and easy – at least in the first semesters – life as students. But then, gradually, steady couples formed, every year I'd get cards proudly announcing marriages or births. Ten years after the *Abitur* exams, there was a class reunion, with a whole host of baby photos to be ooh-ed and aah-ed over.

I was neither one of those who had built a career or had their escapades, nor one of the happy mothers. Of course there were others in the same boat as me, but I had never had anything to do with them in my schooldays and I couldn't rouse any interest in them on this occasion either.

On the day after the reunion, I was no use to anyone. Depressed and ailing, I lay in bed feeling inferior. Very likely I'll not be able to have children at all, I kept thinking. I'm sure I'll try, some day, but it won't work. Shouldn't I at least give it a go, just once? And then? A fatherless child, and no prospects in my job? Very unwise, I told myself, just be patient. In your mid-thirties, there's no need yet for panic about being left on the shelf; these days, a woman can still be young and attractive at forty.

Once, I had this fantastic dream about my own wedding day. I had a door taken off its hinges and a roasted ox served up on it for my father, who never came to see me. My mother, who was compelled to lead an ascetic existence, sat on a barrel like Marlene Dietrich, her legs bared. I sat a nun next to my brother, who had taken a tedious cow for a wife, so that he might get the feeling that he wasn't so badly off with his own dried-up prune after all. As for myself, heavily pregnant, I charged around the astounded company like a flash of ball-lightning.

But who was the fairy-tale prince? Now, more and more frequently, I was dreaming it was Levin.

Frau Hirte had greeted my description of the class reunion with sounds of approval, albeit sleepy ones. Maybe she had drifted off into dreams now and again, who could tell? Sometimes, in the middle of the night, she would suddenly make a grab for her bottle of 'Miss Dior' and douse herself with it. Once I even saw her, since we were never really left in total darkness, sticking the plugs of her walkman in her ears. Very likely, she was listening yet again to her beloved Brahms songs which, like her perfume, she sometimes offered me as others offer you chocolates. Well, it's maybe just as well that she doesn't hear everything, because when you come down to it, I'm talking about things that are really nobody else's business.

3

As part of their prophylactic treatment against possible thrombosis, a good few women have to be mercilessly forced out of bed to be up and about, but not so Frau Hirte. She strides purposefully up and down the corridor, dragging about with her a fair amount of medical luggage in the shape of tubes and bottles. In our time here I have discovered she is quite prudish, and in this regard I try to respect her wishes. Anyway, that suits me much better than the opposite. I have absolutely no time for exhibitionists. Incidentally, she very dutifully wears those horrible white pressure stockings even during the night; me, I'd have them off in a flash.

She doesn't talk much about herself. Mind you, when my former boss came in to see me once, she did get a little bit melancholy. She said she used to take the strain off her own boss, well beyond the call of duty, and what thanks did she get? No sooner had she had to give up work than she had been completely forgotten.

Up till now, I've never been very keen on such confidences between women; all right, I envy my friend Dorit, and in a way she seems quite happy to encourage that. But now, for the first time in my life, I was conscious of a sneaking sympathy for a woman who is a complete stranger, a feeling I had always reserved for men.

I was trying to drive Frau Hirte's cares away with my midnight tales. The next thing she was going to hear about was how Levin and I moved in together.

He came into the chemist's at an unusual time of day for him, even though he knew I didn't like slipping into the back room while my boss was watching.

'What's up?' I asked, looking into a pair of sparkling eyes.
'How would you like to move into a shared flat?' he asked.

Anything but that, was my first reaction. At long last, I had managed to put my own little place straight and keep it free from scroungers, and the only thing I would sacrifice this luxury for was a family of my own. I gave him a firm shake of the head.

'No, wait, let me tell you about it,' pleaded Levin. 'I know of an absolutely regal apartment, just for the two of us, a dream of a place!'

With his beautiful hands, Levin sketched a plan of the place, as accurately as if he were a trained architect.

'No balcony?' I asked in disappointment.

'Not exactly,' said Levin. 'The flat's in Schwetzingen, three minutes from the castle grounds. So you can enjoy your ease like a princess on white benches in the park, admiring the fountains, feeding the ducks, and you can go to all the premières in the Baroque Theatre!'

We rented the big flat in the old block. Through tall lattice windows, the light fell on timbered floors; Tamerlane was able to lead the life of a free tom-cat, climbing up the stems of a clematis in the garden. Yet before long I was missing something else, other than a balcony – my peace and quiet. Up till then, Levin's visits had never lasted more than a few hours, and mostly he didn't stay the night. Now, when I got home, he was always there before me, which by no means meant that the kettle was already whistling. Instead, the radio would be blaring, the television would be on, and Levin would be on the telephone.

'What are we having to eat?' he'd ask by way of a greeting.

Mind you, I myself wouldn't have had it any other way. Naturally, I did his washing, the cooking and the shopping, and I paid the rent. And naturally, he took my car whenever he needed it.

After one particularly strenuous day, I scolded him like some slovenly child. For all that, Levin wasn't really what you would call untidy, it was just that he took up all the space there was. In my two rooms, there were always any number of things lying about which had nothing to do with me, while his room looked almost uninhabited.

'Sometimes you're just like a child,' I said, giving him a kiss.

'Don't you like children, then?' he asked.

I gulped.

'Of course I like children – any normal woman wants children.'

Levin seemed to be thinking things over. 'Would you like to have one?' he asked. He made it sound as if he was about to go out and look for a puppy to go with the kitten.

'In good time,' I said. I didn't want an illegitimate child, but a proper family.

At least once a week, we drove out to see Levin's grandfather in Viernheim. At first I had expected to find him in an old people's home and was amazed to enter a house that was nothing less than a fine villa. The old man lived alone, although he was regularly looked after by an endlessly changing succession of housekeepers. According to Levin, this was on account of his grandad's antediluvian ideas on wages.

Obviously the old man had no conception of present-day prices and was constantly obsessed by the conviction that everybody was out to rip him off. Levin had hardly a good word for him, but he did lavish dutiful care on the house and the garden, drove him to the doctor's and to the bank, and cut his toenails for him. As time went on, I myself took care of things the housekeeper was not in a position to do, typing letters, filling out forms, sorting out laundry and stocking up the freezer. Any other grandad might have expressed his gratitude with more than just the odd dry, blunt word, perhaps a little something now and again. So I considered it all the more to Levin's credit that he went on looking after his grandfather – not without a good grumble now and again.

Once when I was alone with him – Levin had taken the lawnmower to be repaired – I tried to explain to him just what a lousy financial situation his grandson was in.

Hermann Graber (that was the old man's name) looked at me sullenly. 'You think I'm an old skinflint,' he said, rinsing his false teeth unobtrusively (or so he thought) with a mouthful of coffee. 'You've heard I'm rich. But what you probably don't know is that that poor grandson of mine wrote off my new Mercedes. If he starts moaning about having to do a few odd jobs around here for nothing, then I'll leave my money to some orphan instead.'

'That's blackmail,' I thought, with some resentment, as I put a piece of cake on his Alpine-blossom patterned plate.

'And it's also open to question', he went on, 'whether it was the last two housekeepers or my grandson who made off with some gold and silver items . . .'

I flushed and kept quiet.

However, Hermann Graber did not seem to notice, because he had just spotted a black brassière on the washing line in the garden.

On the way home, I pressed Levin for more details of the car accident. He was none too pleased, but he told me the story.

'I was probably overtired and nodded off for a moment. I was on my way back from Spain, you see, and had been flogging on right through the night . . .'

That struck me as highly irresponsible. 'Was anybody hurt?'

'Not exactly. A lorry drove into the Mercedes and its trailer overturned. Guess what he had on board. Jam! Can you imagine what the motorway looked like after that?'

'I asked you if anyone was hurt, not about jam.'

'Actually it was plum jam, to be exact.'

Neither of us spoke for a while.

Levin now had to drive the old man hither and thither, but always at a snail's pace. He was allowed to take the new Mercedes, but never again for his own use.

'So how did your grandad make his fortune?'

'He was an electrician in a small factory, and he invented some kind of intermediate component, I don't know what exactly, which he then manufactured in a works of his own. He made a fortune while still a young man, but later on the firm just bumbled along. When my father died, he sold up.'

I knew that Levin's father had been an organist, with apparently no interest whatsoever in a manufacturing career.

'Your grandfather seems to have definite intentions about your education,' I said, and I couldn't help gloating, just a little.

Levin rejected that. 'He's a sadist who makes me go everywhere by bike! Anybody else would slip the odd thousand into his grandson's pocket now and then.'

We were driving along the autobahn, although I would very much have preferred the romantic Bergstrasse by way of Weinheim. As so often before, it seemed to me that Levin was driving too fast – but this time I got into a real panic about it.

'Slow down a bit,' I pleaded. 'We're in no hurry. Anyway, I think it's very decent of you to go and see your grandfather, even without any reward.'

Levin made no effort to ease off. 'It's certainly not out of any sense of decency that I keep going to see him,' he said. 'As far as I'm concerned, he might as well drop off his perch today as tomorrow, but he's always threatening me with changing his will.'

I couldn't refrain from remarking, 'You haven't actually been doing very much cycling lately. So you can bear to wait quite patiently to come into your inheritance.'

'Till I'm old and grey. That old fellow's clinging on to life, he could reach a hundred!'

I laughed. 'Then let him! Maybe you've got the same genes and you'll live just as long. Anyway, what on earth would you do with the legacy?'

Levin was getting more and more agitated. 'Buy a racing car, travel, enter the Paris – Dakar Rally. I certainly wouldn't have to spend my life pulling rotten teeth.'

I fell silent. Neither the medical profession nor I had any place in his plans.

The next evening, I pointedly left Levin's doctoral thesis lying on the kitchen table and, after weeks of neglect, turned my attention back to my own. I was a stupid fool; the way things were going, I would neither get my doctorate and take up an academic job, nor get married and have children.

So when I then phoned Dorit, I was thoroughly disgusted with myself, but I did confess to her how deeply I had got involved in Levin's career.

'I'm not in the least surprised,' she exclaimed. 'You should never have moved in with him. Do you really love him?'

'I'm pretty sure,' I said.

And that's the way it was. Despite all the reservations my head could come up with, despite all the warning signs that I could almost feel physically, yes, I loved him. Whenever he lay there asleep beside me, curled up like a foetus, I could have wept out of tenderness. Whenever he bolted his food and expressed his delight in my good cooking, when he got all enthusiastic about the little samples from the chemist's, whenever he cheered up in my company, then everything, but everything, was perfect. There were hours of sheer bliss, when we would sit on the sofa with Tamerlane, both stroking him together as we followed James Bond's car chases on the television. But there were also lonely evenings, when I had no idea where he had got to. Naturally, each of us was completely at liberty to come and go as we pleased. I was far too proud to quiz him, perhaps also too afraid of losing him.

When, once again, feeling slightly depressed, I had fallen asleep in front of the television, I was wakened by the phone. Levin, I thought, at last you're learning manners!

'Hella Moormann speaking,' I said.

'Oh, sorry, I must ha' got the wrong number,' said an agitated female voice.

Disappointed, I hung up. A minute later, it was ringing again. It was the same young voice. ''Scuse me. Is Levin there? You 'is girlfriend?'

'Just who is this?' I said coldly, although the voice did seem somehow familiar.

''S me, Margot,' I heard. She was the new, inexperienced housekeeper at Levin's grandfather's. Hermann Graber had had a heart attack, she said, and had been taken to hospital.

She had been told to inform his nearest relatives right away, because his condition was serious.

Now sleep was right out of the question. When, just before midnight, Levin shut the door of the flat behind him – no attempt to sneak in! – he could see straight off that something was bothering me.

'Has the doctor been on the phone?'

'No, his housekeeper, Frau . . . I don't even know the girl's name. She just announced herself with "Margot".'

'That's all we call her,' said Levin.

Naturally, I hadn't imagined he would exactly burst into tears, but I didn't expect such obvious delight either. It was too late to phone again, so Levin said he would drive to the hospital the next morning. 'More important than the university,' he said.

Neither of us slept much. Levin was in bed in the next room, but again and again I heard him getting up, going into the kitchen or the bathroom, switching the radio or the television on and off again. Even I began to picture us living in the lovely villa very soon. And there would be plenty of room for children there.

'Everything's just fine,' Levin declared on his return the next day. 'Grandad was very touched that I was on the spot so soon, but he's in a pretty bad way. The doctor in charge said the end could come quite quickly, his old ticker's not up to it any more. He said they really ought to do a bypass operation, but with an eighty-year-old, that's just not on.'

Then nothing would do but I came to the front door with him, and there stood a Porsche.

'I can have it cheap, and it's nearly new,' he said, in raptures.

'Do you really need it?' I asked.

He looked at me as if I was one spark-plug short of the full set.

I got in to go for a trial spin, with him driving so fast I nearly passed out. And all the while he nagged at me to take out a further bank loan, since the banks were too miserable to lend anything to a student.

I stood firm.

Levin's argument was that he would soon be swimming in money, but this little gem could well have slipped through his fingers by then.

Having such high hopes of the death of a close relative struck me as completely out of order.

The big kid, desperate to have his outsize toy, and to have it now, then resorted to flattery. He praised my proven generosity and dangled the promise of a surprise before me.

I was on the verge of saying, 'Wedding?', but managed to choke the question back. It would have been humiliating if he had then reacted with an incredulous, baffled stare. So I played dumb. 'A holiday?' I asked.

Levin shook his head. 'No use guessing, you'll never get it. You're going to be the architect and interior designer when the villa in Viernheim is renovated.'

Coolly, and without betraying any visible sign of emotion, I said, 'Do you think I have a particular talent in that direction?'

Levin laughed. 'Every woman likes to set up her own home.'

I was so overwhelmed I threw my arms round him. Then I went to the bank to apply for a loan, which was granted, but on very unfavourable terms.

Levin was in seventh heaven and seemed to be out and about in the Porsche from morning till night; it was a good thing the university vacation had just begun.

Hardly had I finished my stint at the chemist's when I would be picked up and whisked off to Frankfurt or Stuttgart, or, at weekends, to the Mediterranean or the North Sea coast. I did have occasional doubts as to whether I had really done him a favour. What if he were to wipe himself out like James Dean, leaving me with nothing but a mountain of debt to remind me of my one and only presentable candidate for marriage?

When, two weeks later, I stood at Hermann Graber's bedside, I did not get the impression I was visiting a dying man. The old fellow was quite chirpy and was making plans.

'If we're lucky,' he said, 'I'll be getting home next week. The doctors are always on at me to take on a nurse, but I'm in no mood to throw good money away unnecessarily. All right, Margot isn't the brightest, but it'll do her no harm to stir herself a bit more.'

After my visit to the hospital, we drove out to the villa and, while Levin mowed the lawn, I had a word with Margot.

'It seems Herr Graber will be coming home soon,' I said. 'Do you think you would manage to nurse him if need be – I mean, over and above the housework?'

'Oh yeah, sure,' said Margot and promptly demanded a raise.

On the drive home, Levin was sullen, to say the least. 'All right, don't say a word,' he barked at me. 'You'll get your money back, don't worry. Who would have thought the old devil could come back from that!'

'Don't trouble yourself, the money can wait. But we're going to have to go out there more regularly when he's back at home. I'm not sure Margot is up to the extra responsibilities. I reckon she's quite unsuitable.'

'Oh, come on, what gives you that idea?' said Levin. 'She's okay. What more do you want for what she's being paid? I even caught Grandad scanning the garden with his binoculars – Margot likes to sunbathe topless, see? I got her for him; the last ones were all useless.'

Then I heard that he had known Margot since primary school days, although she had then gone on to secondary modern, while Levin went to the grammar school. After she had broken off an apprenticeship as a seamstress, she had gone to work in a factory, and then she had been unemployed.

Margot was a chain-smoker and thin as a rake. Some vague hunch made me ask, 'Has she ever been involved with drugs?'

'What makes you think that?'

I had never told Levin anything about my past experiences; Margot fitted exactly into the picture of all those poor wretches I had taken up with. Although they had always been poor men. Where Margot was concerned, it was suddenly quite clear to me: I didn't like her.

My aversion to Margot, although only an indefinable feeling at first, hardened a few days later when Dorit gave me the news (not without a certain smugness) that she had seen Levin getting into a car with a woman. Naturally, I immediately asked what she looked like.

'I'd have credited your sweetheart with rather better taste. The absolute opposite of you.'

Although I already had a pretty shrewd idea that this was Margot we were talking about, I pressed her for a more accurate description.

'Bleached hair, a botched job, with the mousy roots showing through the blonde, dreadfully skinny, about Levin's own age; a poor, common creature.'

That was her, to the life. I couldn't help grinning. The only thing Dorit had omitted to mention was the bitten-down fingernails.

4

It was at my own request that I was put into a surgical ward. The last thing I wanted was to share a room with some mother with her newborn infant at her breast every few hours. I've never been an optimist, and I've already learnt all too often in life that other women's normal happiness is not to be my lot. Yet Frau Hirte contradicted me in this. 'Rubbish,' she said. 'It'll all sort itself out.'

'Dorit has always been a model for me of the way it could be. In contrast to me, she was really loved by her parents, not merely exploited for their own ambitions.'

'Good God,' said Frau Hirte, 'I certainly wouldn't want to change places with your friend. Yesterday, when I saw that worn-out drip of a husband of hers . . . he could easily be her father.'

Naturally, I sprang to Gero's defence. 'Fair enough, young and full of life he isn't. But all in all, she's happily married.'

In Frau Hirte's expression I could read the question, 'And what about you?', but she left it unspoken. She knew perfectly well that I'd tell her the whole story anyway, and that we had plenty of time for that – or at least I did.

Frau Hirte is round the twist. I imagine she must have worshipped her boss in the past the way she does the senior consultant now. Recently, the night sister caught me in mid-narrative and gave me a ticking off. Frau Hirte needed rest, she said. But she was put in her place in no uncertain terms. My room-mate insisted that she slept especially peacefully when there was a monotonous flow of words burbling on beside her. And that flow didn't dry up. This time, it was all about Margot.

There had been a woman in our flat. I could smell it, feel

37

it. The hooks on my coat hangers always hang the one way round, so that, if there was a fire, I'd be able to whip everything out of the cupboard with one single sweep. My mother taught me that kind of orderliness, and I'm very finicky about sticking to it. Both my blue striped and my turquoise summer dresses were hanging the wrong way. I inspected the bathroom next. Of course, Levin's visitor had every right to wash her hands here. (On the other hand, she had no business whatsoever in my wardrobe.) In the toilet bowl lay a cigarette-end, a disgusting habit which, because of the durability of the filter-tips, I cannot abide. Not that this was one of Levin's vices; he emptied his ashtray every day. I had noticed this nasty practice several times already in the villa.

In Levin's room, which I also inspected, there were comics lying about and two empty beer cans on the windowsill. I tried to console myself with the thought that they were just kids. But what, in Levin's case, would evoke no more than a schoolteachery shake of the head, I was not prepared to take from Margot one little bit. She was supposed to be taking over responsibility for caring for a sick old man very soon; she was nothing more than an employee, so what was Levin doing bringing her here? I couldn't bear the smell of her cheap perfume, a synthetic apple-blossom scent.

'Has Margot been here?' I asked when he came home.

He gave me a quick, searching look and decided it was better not to lie. Since, unlike me, she loved fast cars, he said, he had taken her for a spin in the Porsche; after all, we had to keep her in a good mood. I couldn't really see why. But I said nothing about the coat hangers, not wanting to seem like a fussy old thing who, in contrast to young people, didn't like fast driving and was jealous into the bargain. In my nightmares I would see Levin failing to take a bend, but while I was awake I tried to suppress such visions. My constant mothering of my male friends was making me into a perpetual loser.

All the same, Margot had no style whatsoever. I simply could not imagine what the connection was between Levin and her. All right, he came from around here, had close ties with the area and the people, whereas I, an incomer from

Westphalia, had never quite managed to feel at home. With Margot, he always talked in the local dialect, and maybe that gave him a feeling of security. Levin had once spent half a semester at a university in the Ruhr, but since such delicacies as onion tart and pretzel rolls were unknown there, it hadn't been long before he headed back home.

When we brought Hermann Graber back from the hospital, Margot had at least laid out the table for coffee – a rather kitschy arrangement, with three cyclamens in a purple vase placed in front of the convalescent – and had made strong coffee to go with the bought-in cream cake, delights that the ailing grandfather was not allowed. Levin and I ate and drank, so as not to offend Margot, while Grandad demanded a corn schnapps. Without a second thought, Levin brought him his drink. Margot and I had promised Levin not to mention the Porsche, but she almost let the cat out of the bag.

Hermann Graber was clearly delighted to be back in his own home. 'They'll never get me in a hospital again,' he said. 'Your mind just turns to silly things there.'

Politely, I asked, 'For example?'

He laughed. 'For example, that maybe you could change your will!'

Levin went pale. He jumped to his feet and said, 'Come on, Hella. We have to go.'

'What about me wages?' demanded Margot tactlessly.

Grandfather ran a finger over the largest wart on his nose. 'Just so that you don't come up with any daft ideas, you're not going to inherit anything until you've completed your studies. Who knows, I could die tomorrow, and then you'd reckon you wouldn't have to do another hand's turn.'

I felt he wasn't so far off the mark there.

'So what about me wages, then?' Margot asked again.

Although this was far from the appropriate moment, Levin tried to explain to his grandfather: 'Margot should get a raise, Grandad. I mean, everything has got so much more expensive . . .'

'They're all after my money,' said Herr Graber.

For Levin's sake, I added my tuppence-worth.

'So what would you suggest?' the old man asked me directly.

My sense of justice got the upper hand over my aversion; he accepted my suggestion, remarkably without batting an eyelid. Margot didn't go so far as to say 'Thank you', but did manage a 'That's all right, then!'

As we were leaving, he gallantly kissed my hand, getting so excited as he did so that he spilled coffee over himself. I was almost touched. Levin looked on, boiling with rage.

After my discovery that Margot had been here in the flat, I developed a suspicious revulsion at any unusual signs in my rooms. I set traps, stretching a hair over my jewel case, blowing powder across the glass shelves in my bathroom cabinet, marking the level in my perfume bottle and placing a wobbly vase in my wardrobe which would be bound to fall out if the door was jerked open.

For a while, however, there was neither the smell of any female stranger nor the sign of any of my traps being sprung. Perhaps it was all just a distorted product of my imagination and I had hung the coat hangers the wrong way round myself. Too often in the past, I had had to do with shady customers, and I was probably going off my head. It was only my cat who was leaving hairs and footprints around. Yet, one evening, when I carefully opened the cupboard, there was the vase, lying in bits on the floor, and the little brown glass bottles were not in their usual order. Here, too, I had my secret arrangement; the first letters of the individual labels made up the word ANEMONE, but now the letters had been switched around. To my dismay, I read ANOMENE. Levin's looking for the poison, was my first thought, and my stomach churned. I checked the lining of the woollen skirt, but he had found nothing.

The hiding place had been well chosen. Margot was very unlikely to be interested in that old skirt.

Naturally, I wondered whether I should demand an explanation from Levin. My instincts were all against this. That would no doubt mean I had to come out with accusations, suspicions. He would deny everything, and I would be left looking like an avenging schoolmistress. Best just to keep a close eye on him.

My suspicions were reinforced one evening when Levin, the picture of innocence, asked me for something to help him sleep.

'At your age', I said, and startled myself with my maiden-auntish words, 'that shouldn't be necessary. If you don't sleep well two nights in a row, then you'll manage all the better on the third.'

Levin didn't even bat an eyelid. 'Strict Hella,' he said, 'always concerned for my health and my wellbeing. I don't lay much store by pharmacology, I know, but an exception can be made now and again.'

Annoyed, I said, 'If you think you need sleeping pills, then get your doctor to prescribe some.'

That evening, he was noticeably affectionate and attentive, fell asleep in my bed and didn't even wake when I had to leave for work in the morning.

Since Levin was in the habit of making very long calls, my phone often stood in his room. One evening, when I wanted to ring Dorit, I had to go and fetch it. I stopped outside Levin's door when I heard him talking. The key word 'Margot' rooted me to the spot, listening.

'Lawyer? When?' Levin sounded agitated.

On our next visit to Viernheim, I was surprised how healthy and sprightly the old man seemed. He had been put on a new drug for his heart and claimed he felt as if born again. Levin scuttled around the house as if he had to put things straight all over the place.

While this was going on, Hermann Graber took me to one side. 'Is he intending to marry you?' he asked.

I blushed. 'You'd better ask him.'

'It's a comfort to me if that lad is going to be under the wing of a sensible woman. He's a bit irresponsible.'

I nodded, trying to look like a devoted lover.

Hermann Graber explained. 'You remind me a little of

my late wife. My compliments. I'm thinking of changing my will to make it that Levin will inherit only once he has married you.'

'I'd rather you didn't, Herr Graber. Do you think I'd like to get married under pressure?'

Now it was his turn to laugh. 'Giving happiness a little nudge never did any harm. I'm not making any promises, but I'm an old man who finds it fun to play at fate. My lawyer thinks I'm addled, because I'm forever changing my will, but then I keep getting such nice ideas. When Levin wrecked my Mercedes, I offset it against his statutory legacy for the time being.'

His beautifully formed hand, covered with brown age marks, reached out for mine and held it, pleadingly.

'I hope you'll live a long time yet and have lots more fun changing your will,' I said with just a touch of irony. But it didn't faze him.

'I can see we understand each other. I could leave everything to my first grandchild – what do you say to that? That would be sure to have Levin breaking his neck to marry you.'

I found the whole idea very shrewd and very much to my liking, but I dismissed it with a show of modesty.

I told Levin nothing of this conversation; the business with the grandchild was embarrassing. On the other hand, I thought it no bad thing to have a wise old grandfather playing at fate in my favour.

When in doubt, Dorit always said in her blunt way, then keep your hands off. I was always filled with doubts: I seemed to develop a feeling of protectiveness and warmth for my men-friends, but also a sort of sexual dependence on them. I needed their gratitude, their little signs of affection, to feel wanted by them. I didn't want Dorit to get the idea that I always got involved with the wrong kind of men.

I was sitting in her kitchen, telling her about Levin, how hard he was working at his studies, how loyally he was looking after his grandad and, most of all, how happy I was. Dorit listened as she washed a lettuce, cleaned up the sieve and the wooden platter and took crockery out of the dishwasher. Then, her daughter rushed in, crying her eyes out, and at last Dorit sat down. At the sight of that picture of a loving, delicate child being consoled and putting her little arms round her mother's neck, I was again acutely conscious of what I was missing.

'Men are egotists,' said Dorit. 'And we encourage that failing by always putting ourselves second. You're starting to do that even before you're married, and that's not clever. The only reason he's looking after his grandfather is because he's building his hopes on his inheritance – it's all right, I didn't hear that from you, but I do have my other sources – and he's nice to you in order to get everything he can out of you.'

'How do you know about the legacy?' I asked.

'It's no big secret. Gero's from Viernheim and knows the whole story about that old skinflint Hermann Graber, about the collapse of his business and the tragedy of his only son who was determined to become an organist.'

Dorit's husband kept his ears cocked everywhere he went, especially when there was gossip on the go about well-heeled folk. 'Very interesting,' I said. 'So what else has Gero been telling you?'

'The old man was a bit of a rascal, used to get himself driven by taxi once a week to a brothel in Wiesbaden. That hurt his wife very deeply. Now he says he misses her, but there's no doubt he drove her to an early grave.'

'And what's the word about Levin's mother?'

'A woman who got a raw deal. Maybe she's making up for it a bit in her second marriage. Hermann Graber wanted a fine, upstanding man for a son, not a sickly artist; and then his daughter-in-law was to produce a string of grandchildren, but all that amounted to was your Levin, and no doubt all those wishes were projected on to him. Against that, though, the old man never saw him as succeeding to the factory, and as you know, the business was sold long ago.'

'Dorit, would you marry Levin?'

'Of course not, I've got Gero.'

We both had a laugh at that. But then, true to form, she said, 'If you can't be sure, then it's got to be wrong.'

'Oh, Dorit, you married young and you've still got your

43

head full of big ideas. Nothing in life is straightforward, and there are always two sides to everything. But I must say, whenever I see you cuddling your children, then I know that that's exactly what I want.'

'Here you are, go ahead,' said Dorit, plucking the sticky, tear-stained child from her neck and planting her firmly on my lap. While Sarah did sit where she was, she made no effort to cling to me like some sick little monkey.

'Well, cheerio, Dorit,' I said as I finally took my leave and slipped her a packet of Valium I had brought for her. 'Say hello to Gero from me and tell him to be sure to keep his ears open if ever there's any more interesting news.'

I was still on the stairs when I heard the phone ringing. It was a flustered Margot demanding to speak to Levin.

I had no idea when he would deign to come home, I said. Had Hermann Graber taken a turn for the worse?

'Oh, Missis,' she said, and I twitched, 'tell 'im me old man's comin' 'ome.'

When Levin did return, I rather enjoyed passing on the message. 'Her father's coming back.'

Levin shook his head. 'Now she's really going off her trolley. She watches far too many horror films. Her father's hardly going to rise from his grave.' Then he stopped short and asked, to make sure, 'Did she actually say "father"?'

'She talked about her old man.'

He went white and slapped his brow. 'You've misunderstood her altogether. That's not her father, it's her husband!'

'What did you say? – She's married?'

'That's what I'm telling you.'

'And where's the husband been till now?' I had a shrewd suspicion he had been in prison. Naturally I wanted to know why.

'No idea, nothing to do with me,' Levin lied. Then he went into his room to phone. I gave him a couple of minutes before sneaking after him, but all I could catch was the occasional 'I see' and 'Yes, quite right'.

Margot was living at Hermann Graber's, in an extension flat. Would she offer her criminal husband shelter there? That was something I had to prevent at all costs. Heaven knows what kind of a rabble might then be knocking about in our villa. The very thought brought me out in goose pimples. That whole episode in my life with crooks, junkies and neurotics was supposed to be closed once and for all. On the other hand, Margot couldn't be sacked, not just like that. So far, she hadn't done anything wrong and, despite her recent raise, she was still cheap labour.

Levin came back in a bit of a lather. 'She's frightened. But I'm not sure what we can do to help. What do you think?'

'Can't she get a divorce?'

'Then she'd probably feel the real force of his temper. Best thing would be if she could give him some financial support and keep him at arm's length.'

'Does your grandfather know anything about her being married?'

'No, he's never asked.'

Levin was pacing up and down my small living room. There was something else bothering him as well.

'By the way, did you actually throw out that poison?' he asked.

I looked sharply at him. 'Have you been looking for it?'

At last it was all going to come out. 'Do you imagine it's pleasant for me always to be dependent on your money? The old fellow can't be getting much enjoyment out of life any more, and he's going to die sooner or later anyway.'

'Would you mind being rather more precise: what has that to do with the poison?'

'Hella, you know perfectly well what I mean. I've thought of a perfect method. We'd be rid of all our worries. We could live in a lovely house and I could set up a small practice in Viernheim, although I wouldn't have to work myself to the bone, and there would be cash and time to spare for interesting holidays and hobbies – don't you fancy that?'

I was horrified. Barely able to control myself, I said, 'A beautiful dream, but one that can also be realized without committing murder.'

'Who's talking about murder? He's suffering from a decompensated cardiac insufficiency, and his GP knows he could die of it any time.'

'Then wait till that happens.'

'I can't wait any longer. I've got debts.'

These had nothing to do with the Porsche, he said; it was Margot's husband, who was trying to blackmail him. 'He'll do me in if he doesn't get what he wants.'

That cut the ground from under me. Levin, the respectable student from a good home, the first boyfriend with whom there was any prospect of marriage and family life, was mixed up in some dirty business I didn't want to know about. I burst into tears.

Levin took me in his arms, stroking and kissing me. When at last I managed to detach myself from his tear-soaked shirt, I could see that he was looking pretty miserable, too.

'Levin,' I sobbed, 'let's start again from scratch. I'll forget everything you've just told me, and you'll take the cutlery and jewellery back to your grandfather.'

'So that he'll know for sure that it was me. He still thinks it was Margot's predecessor who took it.'

'Just own up and ask his forgiveness.'

'He'd cut me off without a penny.'

'No, he'll forgive a sinner who repents.'

'Never! But, if you insist . . . Where is the stuff?'

I got up and took the gold chain with the Art Nouveau pendant, the green enamelled bracelet and the snake brooch from my jewel case, then went to the kitchen to get the serving fork, the carving knife, the set of fish cutlery and the beautiful teaspoons. I forgot one or two items, but laid all the rest on the table in front of Levin.

'My grandma's dowry,' he remarked as if he were seeing it all for the first time. 'It all belonged to her, not my grandfather.'

I was fiddling with the gold chain, which suited me so well it could have been made specially for me by a goldsmith admirer. What was an old man supposed to do with that? And what good would the exquisite cutlery do him when day in, day out, he got by with a bent fork and a spoon that was practically chewed through? I packed the treasures away again.

5

Whenever he came home from business trips, my father always used to bring back little cakes of soap, shower gel, headed hotel notepaper and tiny packs of butter. Habits like that leave their mark, and I, for my part, have stored away considerable supplies of chemist's samples. Every day here in the hospital, I collect the ready-packed breakfast and supper leftovers, cheese spread, jam, meat paste and even apples and bananas. And Frau Hirte, without a word, deposits what she has salvaged on my bedside table. Recently, Pavel brought all three children with him – pretty late on in the evening, but when you're in the first-class ward they aren't all that strict about visiting hours – and I was able to present them with a bulging bag of groceries.

We were just drinking our red herbal tea. Lene wanted to try some, too, and opened her dainty little mouth wide to get it round the heavy white china. Frau Hirte isn't the least interested in children, so she immediately opened her book. Unfortunately, the two older ones take after their mother very much, although that 'unfortunately' stems from my jealousy, because they are absolutely lovely children. But with the smallest one, my special little darling, it's happily impossible to tell who he takes after.

When my visitors had taken their leave, it still wasn't quite dark. But Frau Hirte said, almost impatiently, 'Let's start a bit earlier today. Maybe I nodded off last night, because I didn't catch why Margot's husband was trying to blackmail your Levin . . .'

Some years previously, Levin and Dieter – Margot's husband, that is – had been arrested at the border between Greece and Turkey. A quantity of heroin was discovered in the heating system of their car, and the vehicle was confiscated. They had agreed beforehand that, in such an event, Dieter would

47

take all the blame on himself, since Levin knew he would be completely and finally cut out of his grandfather's will if he ever fell foul of the law. In return, Levin was to wheedle enough out of the old man to engage a famous lawyer for the defence and, if the possibility arose, to put up bail to get Dieter out. None of this worked out. Hermann Graber wouldn't cough up so much as a single mark, nor did he believe for a moment the tall tale Levin tried to spin him about a total stranger having saved his life by fending off a gang of muggers and landing in prison for his pains, accused of actual bodily harm, when it had been no more than self-defence. 'Surely you don't even believe that yourself,' was all Grandfather Graber had said.

Dieter had got word to Levin that, after having done two years in a Turkish jail, he would be looking for hefty compensation. Nor could he be reasonably expected to wait patiently for Hermann Graber's demise, which could take years.

'Were you on drugs?' I asked. Levin denied it, although he had done a little dealing while still at school, but since this escapade he had steered well clear of them. Dieter, it seemed, was a bit older than him and almost a professional, but he, too, hadn't indulged, other than the odd line of coke (and that only on high days and holidays).

'And what about Margot?'

'Well, yes, she used to, but not any more, I'm sure. I got her the job at Grandad's as proof to Dieter of my good intentions. But I know for a fact he'll blow his top at her starvation wages.'

A starvation wage it certainly was not, but then, after all, Margot was no thrifty housekeeper but a thoroughly incompetent slut. Nevertheless, I was relieved that Levin's association with her was not of an amorous nature.

'Your grandfather's planning for you to come into your inheritance only once you've passed your finals,' I said, 'so it wouldn't make the slightest difference if he died right away.'

'He hasn't been to the solicitor yet,' said Levin, 'so we have to act fast.'

In desperation, I cast around for other arguments. 'You're

not going to prevent a criminal going on blackmailing you, even if you pay up the amount he wants.'

'Dieter's not like that,' Levin contradicted me. 'Even among dealers, there's a code of honour. He'll never shop me, just give me such a beating he'd maim me for life.'

'Sell the Porsche,' I suggested. 'If you're lucky, he'll be satisfied with what you get for it.'

'Okay,' he said. 'Obviously, you'll be happy with a husband you have to scrape off the walls with a fish-slice.'

I was near the end of my tether and snapped back, 'Fine, then give this awful Dieter the poison!'

Levin sucked his teeth. He came up with all sorts of excuses, the main one being that his perfect ploy couldn't work with younger people. Besides, he didn't exactly seem to hate Dieter, while he would happily have strangled his grandfather with his own hands.

For me, it was precisely the other way round.

When I had reached this explosive stage of my story, I turned anxiously to look at Frau Hirte. She was already asleep, so I could quite safely carry on.

Levin finally let me in on his ingenious plan, which depended completely on the tiny poison pills. I had to admit that there was no great risk involved. My fear of being implicated as an accomplice gradually diminished. But my revulsion and my moral scruples were harder to shake off. While I did see that an old man with a heart ailment no longer had much in the way of life expectancy, still, no one had the right 'to play at fate a little', as Levin, and indeed his grandfather, called it.

Levin went on, offering further considerations, 'He won't suffer any pain, he'll die in a matter of seconds, the GP is prepared for his death and will make out the death certificate without looking for any unnatural causes. In any case, I know his doctor, and he's no longer in the first flush . . . Of course, it mustn't happen at a weekend, because then some other emergency doctor would be called in, and there's no telling how he might react.'

I couldn't help thinking of the people in my circle of friends

49

and relations who had hoped for a quick end, dropping dead, with no hospitals, no tubes, no machines. Would Hermann Graber not be better served by this painless demise than having to put up with months of suffering?

'And Margot? What if she notices something?'

'Oh, her! Don't worry, her gifts certainly don't lie on an intellectual level. She knows his heart's bad. When she finds the body, she'll scream and shout and then call the doctor, as is only right and proper.'

'But then there's her husband. Won't Dieter put two and two together if your grandfather dies at such an opportune moment? And anyway, why is Margot so afraid of him?'

'She's got good reason to be frightened. She's been cheating on him, not only with his best friend, but also with his own brother. Dieter will soon find out about all that. But he won't give a hoot what Grandad dies of. All he wants is money, and then we're quits.'

For me, it was all still something of an intellectual exercise when we had another look at the various phials of poison. Levin consulted a medical handbook whenever I wasn't sure, and then he made his choice.

'Do you think the poison will still work?' he asked. 'Maybe we should test it out first,' and his eye fell on Tamerlane.

At that, I almost lost control, but he said quickly, 'Come on, only joking.'

'After preparing a cavity, I'll put in a temporary filling,' he pontificated.

Although I knew perfectly well, I asked (because I loved it when Levin did his academic act), 'What's a cavity?'

'A defect in the enamel of the tooth,' said Levin, revelling in the fact that his umpteen semesters of dentistry studies were proving of some use at last.

My eye fell on the beautiful photo of the grandparents' villa that Levin had hung in the kitchen. This mute picture convinced me much more than all his eloquent pleadings. That's where I belonged, not in some rented flat with no balcony and no garden. Dorit's new house (much more expensive than originally planned) wouldn't be able to hold a candle to it.

* * *

'Just a trial run,' said Levin as we drove out to Viernheim one Thursday evening in the convertible, because the Porsche would attract too much notice.

Hermann Graber was in the habit of going to bed very early, and, nevertheless, getting up late. As he lay in bed, he would watch the entire television programme right through, and, because he was hard of hearing, he always used headphones. This had the advantage that he couldn't pick up other noises about the house, short of a bomb going off. He had no fear of burglars, since all his cash and shares lay in a safe deposit at the bank.

The house was furnished in a style of solid, massive awfulness. Grubby velvet curtains at the doors, carved oak cabinets, panelling blackened with age. Obviously, the old man missed neither his wife's silver caskets nor her porcelain figures, since he couldn't abide dust-traps.

Of course, Levin had a key. 'I've got to do some soldering in the cellar,' he explained to Margot, who was staring inquisitively at the car radio tucked under his arm. Downstairs, Hermann Graber kept an old-fashioned but superbly equipped workshop.

While I worked out a diet for Grandad with Margot in the kitchen, Levin went out to the car to get his dentist's rose-head drill, which he had bought second-hand some time before.

He slipped upstairs with it and took Hermann Graber's set of dentures from its dish, for he knew that his grandfather put his false teeth in water with a cleansing tablet only once a week, on Saturdays, when he also took his bath. On weekdays like this, they would be lying dry in their small bowl on top of the bathroom radiator.

With his special drill, Levin bored tiny holes in two of the artificial teeth around the molar area, just big enough to accommodate one poison pill in each. After he had embedded the dose, he covered them with an extremely thin layer of a dressing for temporary fillings, which would dissolve on contact with saliva.

After the job was completed, he laid the dentures back in the jam-dish and packed the drill and the radio away in the car. When he came to join us in the kitchen, he looked greatly relieved.

'That's the radio working again,' Levin said to Margot. 'Have you heard anything from Dieter?'

'Nothin'.'

'So he could turn up on the doorstep any day?'

'Then Gawd 'elp us!' she said.

We told her we were off to the cinema, and left.

In Heidelberg, we walked along the main street so that we might meet people we knew – which worked out nicely – had an espresso at a café on the Theaterplatz and went into the late showing after it had started, so as to draw attention to ourselves.

Only after the film – of which I can remember nothing – did Levin reveal to me that our visit to the villa had by no means been the dress rehearsal. I burst into tears right in the middle of the street.

That night, we lay together in my bed, endlessly tossing and turning, unable to sleep. Suddenly, I got up and dressed. 'Come on, Levin, we're going to go straight back there and undo the whole thing!' I ordered. Thanks to his overpowering caresses and my sheer exhaustion, however, we did no such thing.

I had to start work at the chemist's at eight, and Levin was to phone me the moment he had any news from Viernheim. He did not rise until somewhat later, let himself be seen in the garden with the cat, went to the pillar box, then to buy a paper and made sure he exchanged good-mornings with neighbours.

'You're coming down with something, Hella,' said my boss. 'I can tell from the look of you.'

I assured her that I was just having my period, when I always looked like death. At that word, I choked and wheezed like an asthmatic.

My boss gave a disapproving shake of the head. 'I think you'd best go home,' she advised. 'It doesn't make the best of impressions on the customers if they catch something from the chemist.'

'It's nothing, really,' I said, almost pleading. 'If it's all right by you, I'll just lie down for ten minutes in the back room.'

I took advantage of this short break to do up my face carefully. It was almost eleven o'clock by then. Maybe, I thought, the poison has lost its effect after all these years. I fervently hoped so.

Just as I was returning, rosy-cheeked, to the counter, the phone rang. Levin said, stiffly, 'I'm afraid I have to deliver the sad news that my grandfather has died. I'll probably call again later. For the moment, I've got to get over to Viernheim at once.'

Every bit as formally, since my boss was eavesdropping, I said, 'Good heavens! Oh, I am sorry! When did it happen? Did the housekeeper call you with the news?'

'No, it was the doctor himself. See you later.'

'Is something wrong?' my boss was eager to know.

I nodded. 'My boyfriend's grandfather has died. But he was old and in poor health, and it was only to be expected.'

'Do you want to leave early?' she asked.

'Thanks very much, but that won't be necessary.'

All that day, there was no more word from Levin. I kept making mistakes in my work, mislaying medicines and forgetting to send out tablets to a sick woman. Punctually, but not a minute early, I left the chemist's shop.

The flat was deserted. At last, at eight, the phone rang. I rushed to pick it up, and it was Dorit. 'I suppose you already know you have a filthy rich boyfriend?' she asked with total lack of respect. 'His grandpa died today.'

'How do you know that?' I asked slowly.

'From Gero. Men are such terrible old gossips. Old Graber's neighbour had seen the hearse outside . . . He's a colleague of Gero's . . . Well, so what's it to be? Are you going to move into the house in Viernheim and disturb the peace with the noise of builders?'

'Questions, questions,' I said tersely. I wanted to keep the line clear for Levin.

'I bought myself a silk blazer today,' Dorit went on. 'Guess what colour! Pink!'

I wasn't in the mood for a chat, so I made my excuses and hung up. I would have loved to take a shower, I was bathed in sweat. But I knew that, the very moment the warm water started to stream over me, the telephone would ring. By this time, it wasn't Levin I was expecting to hear from, but the police, telling me he had been arrested.

At half past eight I heard the Porsche at long last. I ran to the front door and saw an enormous dent in its wing. Levin picked up several plastic carrier bags from the front seat, handed one to me and said, charmingly, 'Your mouth's as wide open as the door! Everything's hunky-dory!'

We had hardly got back into the flat when my nerves went.

But Levin just laughed. 'You're about to see – our waiting has not been in vain!' He unpacked champagne, my favourite salad, fresh shrimps, exotic fruits and crispy vol-au-vents. 'Aren't you hungry?'

Nothing had been further from my mind than eating, but at the sight of all this, my appetite was stirred despite myself. Nevertheless, I wanted to know where he had got to.

'What's with "got to"?' Levin defended himself. 'I've been hard at work the whole time.'

While I brought plates and set out the food, he told his story. Margot had made breakfast at ten that morning; Hermann Graber seemed to enjoy it and, as usual, read the paper as he drank his coffee. When he had finished, Margot went shopping. She was back in half an hour, to find the dead man sitting peacefully at his desk, his playing cards for a game of patience had slipped from his hand. He was still warm, Margot had said, but she got a scare that curled her toenails. She phoned Dr Schneider right away. When the doctor saw nothing more could be done, he made out the death certificate and called Levin. Arriving at Viernheim, Levin was met at the door by a hysterical Margot. It was all her fault, she said, the old man wasn't supposed to drink strong coffee. Levin gave her the rest of the day off.

'And what did you do then?'

'As I said, worked myself to a frazzle. But it's been worth it!'

I didn't quite get the point, but Levin fed me a forkful of shrimps and beamed at me. He refilled his champagne glass. 'Cheers, Hella. Here's to the good times!'

He opened the next carrier bag and dug out a little jeweller's ring-box. 'I reckoned yellow topaz would go well with your brown eyes.' Then he unpacked silk shirts for himself, silk blouses for me, shoes, perfume and a globe of the world.

He had spent ages opening Hermann Graber's safe; Levin had assumed his grandfather would keep some ready cash about the house. The safe was a plain, simple model, no key, just a combination lock. But there had been nothing special in it – personal identity papers, a book with family records and legal documents, and some communications from the bank regarding various deposits, none of them involving great amounts, however.

Levin had then made a systematic search of the bedroom, convinced that that was where the treasure was buried. But it was some hours before he met with any success. 'The old fellow wasn't stupid,' he acknowledged with some admiration. 'Nobody else would have hit on that hiding place.' From a hatch giving access to a chimney flue hung a tiny piece of string. Levin had taken off the wallpaper covering and raised the hinge to reveal a plastic bag with several thousand-mark notes. Of course, this wasn't the much-vaunted legacy, but still something of an advance on the joys to come. Then Levin had called the undertakers and made all the arrangements for the funeral, and after that had tried, without success, to contact the lawyer. Just before closing time, he had done a bit of shopping.

With that, my composure disintegrated. I howled my head off and clung to Levin like a wet rag.

He stroked me. 'It's all right now, it's all over. Come on, lie down and have a sleep, you're badly in need of it. I've got to stay up a while and do a bit of planning.'

After a relaxing herbal bath and a couple of valerian tablets, I dozed off into dreamlike visions. 'As of tomorrow,' I thought, 'I'm off the pill. And it's not as if the ring had anything to do with the old man dying. Levin certainly didn't inherit meanness from his grandfather, but let's hope he doesn't swing to the other extreme . . . I'll just have to educate him a little . . .'

The next morning, I went off to work, while Levin drove out to Viernheim. He had spent almost all the money out of the secret hiding-place.

Should we dismiss Margot? Not for the moment. Levin was against it in the meantime, reckoning it was better for the villa to remain occupied. We weren't going to move in until the place had been completely renovated. Besides, the house was big enough for a dentist's practice to be installed on the ground floor, and that had to be thought out before work started. I was relieved that Levin was thinking ahead so sensibly and not going straight out to buy another car. And, by the way, where did the huge dent come from? Oh, I wasn't to concern myself about that, he had replied, nobody had seen it happen.

Levin was in a desperate hurry to get an appointment with the lawyer. Until then, he could have no idea how much money he could reckon with, or whether the will might not contain some spiteful clause or other. One thing was sure, the villa was worth a dozen Porsches, he assured me, for that was Levin's currency.

The grumpy lawyer made things as tense as he could. The will had in fact been revised twelve times in all, he said. The most recent version was no more than two weeks old, and he himself was unaware of its contents. Levin went white. But there was no mention of his examinations. Levin got some security bonds, which apparently just covered his statutory portion. The villa and the lion's share of the stocks and shares fell to me, Hella Moormann, provided I married Levin within six months. Naturally, I was free to reject both the legacy and marriage if I wished, in which eventuality the fortune would go to the Red Cross.

It took Levin a few moments to digest this message properly.

When the penny had finally dropped, he leapt to his feet, yelling, 'Well, anyone can see the old man was no longer in his right mind! This is sheer madness – a strange woman is to get all the money! Can't he be declared incapable of managing his own affairs, posthumously?'

My scrap of new-found faith and happy anticipation was gone in a flash. The money was the last thing on my mind.

'Legal incapacitation . . .' replied the lawyer, savouring his words, 'that's something that dissatisfied dependants come up with again and again, sometimes even with success. But in your grandfather's case, I see little prospect of that, since he was, right up to the end, in full possession of his mental faculties, as the saying so nicely goes. And there are many people who will testify to that.'

Levin was getting a grip on himself again. 'It doesn't really matter all that much,' he said, fighting to keep his temper. 'My fiancée and I were planning on getting married soon anyway.'

'Well, there we are now, there's nothing standing in the way of the happy ending,' said the lawyer with unconcealed envy as he gave me a smarmy smile. I neither returned his smile nor confirmed Levin's statement. I was deeply hurt.

6

'Did you have a good night's sleep?' I asked Frau Hirte the next morning, for her face had taken on a weary, leaden kind of expression.

She had had a frightful nightmare, she replied; maybe it was the full moon that was to blame.

'So what did you dream about?' I asked apprehensively.

'In my dream, I shot a policeman.'

The very thought of this dried-up, nippy old cow pointing a gun at a policeman made me smile. 'We'll have a look in our Freud, to see what significance that might have,' I suggested.

But she merely asked, 'Have you never had dreams like that?'

I shook my head, too firmly, if anything.

'I was thinking of the business with your classmate,' she went on. 'I mean, something like that just never lets you go as long as you live.'

She was certainly right there.

Unlike me, Frau Hirte had already been in hospital several times. A few years before, she had had an operation on her intestines; she keeps on steadfastly insisting that that finally conquered her cancer. However, the histological results have still to be confirmed, and I reckon the doctors will give it to her straight. Even to a layman, looking at her lying there, all skin and bones, pallid and with no appetite, things would seem pretty gloomy.

'How far did I get yesterday?' I asked, just to test her out.

She was rather at a loss. 'I think you were at the bit about working out a diet for the grandfather,' she said. 'I might have nodded off at that point. Once I got myself a microwave, I packed in cooking altogether . . .'

'Right, fair enough,' I said. 'Grandfather died.'

*   *   *

Hermann Graber's death made me think back to my own grandfather. In all likelihood, I had chosen my profession in an effort to emulate him. Otherwise I would probably have gone in for something like social work, or become a psychologist or a doctor, a nursery-school teacher or a nurse – just as well things didn't turn out that way; my personal life would always have come a hopeless second. As a pharmacist you certainly have to deal with people who are suffering, true, but at least, most of them leave the shop without having emptied their emotional dustbin on you every time.

My grandfather was a handsome, white-haired patriarch, widely respected and highly regarded. Like Hermann Graber, he had put together a tidy fortune, but I, unlike Levin, was very attached to my grandfather, and, every time I shared Grandad's armchair with Tamerlane, I would think back on him with affection. If anyone had even thought of doing away with my grandfather, I would have detested that person for the rest of my days.

After Levin had reacted so obnoxiously to the will, my feelings for him cooled off. On the drive home from the lawyer's, he asked, 'What's up? Why have you gone so monosyllabic? After all, you've good reason to be happy: you, the outsider, you've won the game.'

I neither regarded our deed as a game, nor did I see myself as the victor. 'Just you wait, my lad,' I thought. 'You won't catch me that easily.'

Naturally, it was not long before he asked when the wedding was to take place.

'Don't know,' I replied coldly.

'In theory, we've got six months to play with,' said Levin. 'But Dieter could show up any day, so we really should get a move on.'

'Get a move on? What for?' I asked. 'If you sell your shares or the Porsche, you can pay him off.'

His jaw dropped.

'So that's the way it is, then,' he said. 'I'm to shell out while you settle down at your ease on my fortune.'

'Until we're married, not a penny of it's mine,' I exclaimed.

'You know that perfectly well. And you also know that I'm not money mad.'

Levin looked at me as if I had grown a second head. 'Is that supposed to mean that you don't want me any more and you'll let the legacy go down the drain? We could always get divorced; I mean, let's face it, it would be a shame if the Red Cross just copped the lot.'

'I've got nothing against the Red Cross,' I retorted.

Levin burst out laughing. 'Madam will have her little joke,' he said, making a grab at me.

I remained stiff as a board. 'No kissing strange women,' I warned.

Then he caught on. 'The wedding's on – in a week!' he proposed, just like that, but I kept stubbornly silent.

For the next few days we left each other to stew, each waiting for peace offerings from the other.

Nor did the famous Dieter put in an appearance. From time to time I had doubts about his existence, even though Margot had got into such a lather about him coming back. Once, I even had my suspicions that Levin and Margot had invented this ghost from the past. But I rejected this thought, for Levin would never make common cause with that stupid bitch. Well, yes, he was irresponsible, but no schemer.

It was Levin who gave in, in the end. He came to collect me in the Porsche, even though my convertible was standing outside the shop, and suggested we go somewhere expensive for a meal.

'So, are you determined to blow your money straight away?' I asked.

He didn't so much as blink, but all the same I knew that any reference to thrift was like a red rag to a bull for him. 'We haven't celebrated our engagement yet,' he said.

I wanted to go home first to have a shower and change.

Once we were finally ensconced in the restaurant, I sank back exhausted into the plush upholstery, drank some wine and eased myself out of my intransigence.

Levin had set it all up very cleverly. After a few glasses, probably two more than was good for me, he asked boldly, 'If you had one wish, what would it be?'

'A child.'

The next day, we published the announcement of our forthcoming marriage. It was a Saturday, and my day off, but I didn't want to go shopping with Levin and got on with some cleaning instead. Would we, I wondered, soon be able to take on a cleaning woman?

The doorbell rang. Dorit, I thought, and at a bad time. Whenever she was in the house, we were bound to spend hours talking about men and children.

However, it wasn't Dorit but a fine, strapping man I found on the doorstep. 'Does Levin Graber live here?' he asked, rather uncertainly, even though the nameplate made it quite clear.

No, I didn't know when Levin would be back; but he said he'd wait all the same.

'My name is Dieter Krosmansky.'

I jumped.

Dieter seemed to be watching me closely. 'If it doesn't suit, I can come back this evening.'

'Damn,' I thought, 'he can tell I know who he is, and he thinks I've got a thing against people just out of prison.'

So I invited him in, ever so nicely, showed him into Levin's room and brought him the paper and a beer. I left the door open. I was rather afraid Dieter might rummage about in Levin's things. Duster in hand, I walked determinedly into the room, made my apologies and started dusting around Dieter. We each watched the other out of the corner of an eye. With feigned cheerfulness, I asked whether he was a native of Heidelberg.

'No, but I used to live here. My family comes from the East.'

Dieter spoke very correct German, not like Margot, who could never have concealed the fact that she came from this area. Was he really her husband? Getting on with

61

my polishing, I asked, all bright and innocent, 'Were you at university with Levin?'

'Not exactly,' said Dieter, just as nicely. 'But we have done a bit of travelling together.'

Well, now we were getting closer to the heart of the matter already. Dieter seemed to be trying to work out whether I was just a passing fancy or a steady girlfriend, and whether I was in the know about Levin's past.

I helped him out. 'Levin and I are getting married very soon,' I said.

'Can I take it, then, that Levin has finished his studies?'

'Not long now, and he will have.'

'By the way, is his grandfather still alive?'

That was the sixty-four-thousand-dollar-question, but there was no point in playing the innocent on that one. 'He died just recently.'

'Well, so Levin must be a rich man now. I'm surprised that, in these circumstances, he's happy to make do with just the one room.'

'He's trying to sound me out,' I thought, annoyed with myself. Served me right. 'The will comes into force only once it's gone through the probate court,' I said, 'and these things take time.'

He didn't follow up the point, but suddenly said, 'I don't feel too good. Do you think I might lie down for a while? I'm sure Levin won't mind if I just stretch out for a rest on his bed.'

Reluctantly I watched him taking off his shoes (which was something, at least) and settling down; all that was holding the thinner parts of his socks together was the nylon ribbing. With an uneasy feeling, I made my exit, leaving the door slightly ajar.

When I had polished the whole flat till it was gleaming, Levin had still not come back and Dieter was still sound asleep. I crept over to his bed and had a good look at him. He didn't fit my picture of a drug dealer; that wasn't what villains looked like. In his checked shirt and corduroy trousers he reminded me more of a British student or a Westphalian land surveyor. His face bore all the signs of total exhaustion;

all in all, an intelligent face, one which, if I were to be honest, I found not altogether unattractive. How on earth did he land up with Margot! It somehow moved me to see that the nail on his left thumb was deformed. I found myself feeling almost sorry for this sleeping man, so I fetched a woollen rug from my room and spread it over him.

Because he had bought something special to eat, Levin was not all that late in getting home. I sneaked to the door when I heard the car pulling up and opened it before he could get his key in the lock, put a finger to my lips and whispered, 'He's here!'

'Who?' Levin asked, much too loudly.

I gestured to him again to be quiet and led him to his bed. Incredulous, Levin stared at his old mate and then followed me into the kitchen. My brave little friend was on edge, playing with his cigarettes and wanting to know what we had talked about.

'Don't worry, he was as gentle as a little lamb,' I said. 'But I had to tell him your grandfather was dead. He'd have found out anyway.'

Levin was jumpy. 'What are we going to do with him now?'

'Let him sleep, have a meal with him and go for a stroll in the castle gardens,' I suggested.

Levin gawped at me. 'Who would have thought you'd keep your cool like this? You'd have made a great gangster's moll!'

I stopped myself saying that I had already been through that and started preparing the meal, while Levin, prowling about restlessly, kept getting in my way. As a therapeutic diversion from his agitation, I gave him some apples to peel. Levin picked up the sharpest knife we had, and promptly cut his fingers. As I was putting on a bandage our visitor, still in his socks, suddenly appeared before us. At the sight of the drops of blood he went white and turned away. I wiped the table clean.

Dieter approached again. 'Well, how's it going, old mate?' he said, slapping Levin heartily (a bit too heartily?) on the back. 'Isn't Margot living in Heidelberg any more? At Lore's place in the Grabengasse?'

Levin was evasive. 'Hella's an excellent cook if she's left in peace. Come on, we'll have a drink first.'

The pair of them disappeared, while I got on with braising the rabbit in the frying pan along with some grapes from which I had laboriously removed the pips, slices of apple and some Calvados. Not a word got through to me.

When, half an hour later, I announced dinner was served, I found the two men in the best of spirits, with no sign of any physical or verbal dispute having taken place.

The rabbit had turned out a success, and both lavished praise on it. We chatted about politics, gossip and recipes. Until Dieter abruptly got to his feet and said, 'Give me your car. You'll get it back tomorrow.'

I was completely taken aback by this demand and couldn't imagine Levin ever letting the keys to his Porsche out of his possession. There was a slight twitch at the corners of his mouth, and he said, 'I'll drive you.'

'Nice of you to offer, but absolutely unnecessary,' said Dieter. 'You've had more to drink than I have.'

That certainly was true. Levin handed over the keys. 'You know where to find it, I'm sure.'

The moment he was gone, I asked, 'Is he going to Margot? Will he beat her up? What does he want from you?'

Levin yawned. 'My treasure, as you may have noticed, Saul has become Paul. We got along fine, and he won't touch a hair of Margot's head.'

'And what about the money you owe him?'

'That can wait,' said Levin. 'Oh, by the way, he's going to be our best man.'

That was not at all to my liking, for it meant that, like it or lump it, Margot would be at our wedding. I had invited my parents, whom I visited only rarely now, and my brother, as well as, of course, a few friends and my boss. I had intended Dorit and Gero to be the witnesses, now it was to be Dorit and Dieter. For years on end, my parents had got upset about my questionable lovers, and now they were at last supposed to have the satisfaction of seeing their daughter marrying a

64

suitable academic with a considerable inheritance. If Margot were to turn up, the good impression would in all certainty be shattered.

Levin laughed at my misgivings. 'I'd never have imagined you to be so snooty! But you apparently have no objection to Dieter?'

I didn't say a word. But I had to admit to myself that Dieter might even create a better impression on the impartial observer than Levin himself. 'How old is Dieter? Does he have a job?' I asked.

'Mid-thirties, thereabouts, and he did take some course or other, insurance salesman, I think. He's a clever bloke, can speak several languages.'

'So why should such a clever bloke get into drug dealing?'

'A good question, I'll grant you that. But what won't people do for money?'

I wanted to stash my little tubes of poison away somewhere else. It wasn't right for a rash, unthinking person like Levin to continue to have access to them. While I was searching around for a safe hiding-place for them, I tried to figure out why my grandfather had hoarded such dangerous poisons, apparently of British origin. Things like that most certainly did not form part of the standard equipment in any chemist's, as I had pointed out to Levin. Did it have something to do with the fact that, in the Third Reich, Grandfather had been mixed up in some things my family never talked about? I put the poison into an old flowerpot, tipped soil in on top of it and placed the pot in the cellar, alongside other bits and bobs that had once graced my former balcony. The day of the wedding was getting close. I was in a tizzy, there were so many things to be worked out. What was I going to wear? Dorit came with me to buy a cream-coloured linen suit. For a bouquet, she suggested pink moss-roses, lilies and forget-me-nots. But I reckoned that would make me look too pale.

Levin had other things on his mind. 'Come on,' he said, three days before the big event, 'we're going to drive out to Viernheim, I know an architect there. We'll have to get down to giving some thought to what's to be done with the house.'

So it was that I came back to the villa for the first time after Hermann Graber's death. The huge rooms on the ground floor, which had previously remained darkened and unused, suddenly looked altogether different: Dieter and Margot had rearranged the heavy, black furniture and made themselves at home there. Apparently Margot had moved out of her basement room and into the grander family apartments. The sight filled me with foreboding.

The architect put forward suggestions as to how the old house could be modernized and renovated without ruining its character. I wanted to have a conservatory built on. But before anything was done, it had to be decided whether the ground floor was to be used for the dental practice; if so, a separate entrance could be included in the plans. Levin, rather lukewarm, said he hadn't made up his mind yet.

Once the architect had gone, Dieter brought some wine from Hermann Graber's cellar. Since he was to be our best man, he said, we should all get on first-name terms at last. Raising his glass, he said, 'Here's to you, Hella!'

I had been caught completely unawares; now I even had to put up with Margot, who had until then, on my insistence, always addressed me as 'Frau Moormann', calling me 'Hella'. I was annoyed with myself for my reluctance especially since I had always been critical of my parents on account of their snobbishness.

'I'm not at all happy', I told Levin on the drive home, 'with the idea of your lot simply taking over the house in Viernheim. My parents and your mother could have stayed the night there.'

'I haven't even been able to get in touch with my mother,' said Levin.

That made me even more discontented. It was a matter of good form for both sets of parents to be present. I changed the subject. 'Can you explain to me just why Dieter came to marry that stupid tart of all people?'

'A tart like that is by no means something to be sneezed at. She once helped him out of a tough spot.'

'That's no reason to go and marry her right off; they're not in the least suited to each other.'

'And how are you supposed to be the judge of that?' said Levin.

7

'Were you really so stupid as to actually marry that waster?' demanded Frau Hirte. 'If so, then please skip the wedding, if you don't mind, and go straight on to the successful divorce proceedings.'

Obviously she had been listening attentively to the last part. But the wedding was important, and I couldn't simply pass over it.

We were interrupted by the doctor's rounds. Once again, with his usual outrageous lack of tact, Dr Kaiser hoicked up Frau Hirte's bedclothes and nightdress to scrutinize the state of her scar. He seemed satisfied, gave her slack stomach a few pokes and asked whether she had taken any hormone preparations while she was going through the menopause.

'After the operation on Frau Hirte's colon, hormones were contra-indicated,' said the ward sister, rolling her eyes heavenwards at the doctor's forgetfulness. He merely reached out his great paw to shake my hand, saying he would be seeing me again shortly at the ultrasound scan.

It was not until evening that things had returned to peace and quiet enough for me to give Frau Hirte the benefit of the next instalment of my life story.

During the wedding preparations, Dorit proved once again to be a real friend. She helped me with all the organizing, booked hotel rooms, set her mind to the table decorations and gave mutual friends tips for suitable presents. Levin had little or no interest in such things, but he did consult the head chef in the Castle Restaurant in Schwetzingen and drew up a princely menu for the wedding meal.

*   *   *

A day before the great event, I was once more sitting in Dorit's kitchen, cooling my tired feet in a basin of water laced with fragrant essences to perk up my circulation. I felt so close to her at that moment that, quite contrary to my intentions, I told her all about how the sizeable inheritance would soon be mine and not Levin's after all. At that, she pricked up her ears. She wanted me to promise her never to grant Levin power of attorney over my fortune – she wouldn't put it past him to have blown the lot within a year.

I made a feeble attempt to object. 'But Dorit, he'll insist on it. And anyway, I've never been very materialistic in outlook . . .'

She became sarcastic. 'I know, I know, for you it's only a person's inner values that count. All the same, for the old man it was vital that somebody kept an eye on the precious Levin. He trusted you, otherwise he'd never have changed his will in your favour.'

I had to admit she was right, and promised to exercise caution.

My brother, along with his wife and child, was expected from down south, while my parents would be coming down from the north. When they arrived, Levin was not at home; he wanted to give me the chance to be alone with them all. My parents' prejudices against their future son-in-law, whom they hadn't even met yet, were written all over their faces.

It was my mother who came out with the standard question: 'What did his father do for a living?'

'Organist.'

'You mentioned something about a legacy. But surely, a church mouse . . . ?'

'The inheritance comes from his grandfather.' I could read the question, 'How much?' in my parents' expressions, but of course they were much too refined to come straight out with it.

My father went snooping round our flat, surveying it for neatness and cleanliness. Without so much as a by-your-leave, he also had a good look round Levin's room. At last, he spoke up. 'How old is he?'

'Twenty-seven.'

He sighed. Thirty-seven would have been more to his liking. He was stirring the tea in his cup incessantly, even though he had given up taking sugar more than twenty years before.

Thankfully, my brother brought a breath of fresher air with him. His tedious wife had stayed behind in the hotel with the child. I always had the feeling that she rejected me. Bob hugged me and my parents and assured me of how happy he was that I was getting married.

Much to my relief, when Levin arrived, the conversation turned to neutral topics, and we ended up on the subject of cars.

My parents were watching their son-in-law with grim attentiveness, without however being immediately able to find any fundamental objections to him. For the very first time, I noticed that Levin always left the top three buttons on his shirt undone. The evening passed amicably enough, and my family retired early to their hotel beds.

The day of the wedding began with glorious weather, and my parents were in a reasonably good humour. With a conspiratorial expression on her face, my mother drew me into the kitchen and gave me a present of a dozen snow-white hotel bath-towels, the product of the twelve business trips on which Father had taken her along in the course of their married life.

After a rather heavy breakfast, prepared by my stout mother and my skinny sister-in-law, the witnesses came to pick us up. Dorit and Dieter both acted very responsibly and extremely nicely, so that I had nothing to be ashamed of in front of my parents. In any case, it wasn't as if they didn't know Dorit already, and indeed they considered her to be a good influence on me. After the civil wedding, we all gathered again in the coffee-room in the Castle. I looked so pretty, or at least so I imagined; my costume suited me perfectly and my father had put round my neck, with his own fair hand, the six rows of polished pearls and garnets which had belonged to his grandmother and which I had had my eye on for a long time.

But then it all started to go wrong. I caught sight of Margot and was horrified. Was this the mangy cat that had, after a fashion, taken care of Hermann Graber's household? Before me stood a young woman in a black dress, the top half transparent and, at the back, plunging all the way down to the start of the valley between her buttocks; totally out of place, and no doubt paid for out of my money. And, confronted with this concentrated package of aggressive low-class sex, many of the men were asking eagerly, 'Who's that, then?'

Fortunately, at the meal, Margot was seated well away from me. But my brother immediately moved over next to her and seemed to be having a good time.

Next to my boss (in a kiwi-coloured safari dress) sat Hermann Graber's old family physician, Dr Schneider. Levin had invited him on the pretext that it was a good move to keep in with a future colleague. I had had no objection to that. There were other Viernheim dignitaries present, too. After all, we were intending to live in the town in the near future, and sooner or later Levin would be setting up his practice.

After the coffee, a dance-band arrived. Up till then, Levin had never danced with me, claiming he had never mastered the art. The band was Dieter's wedding present, and it pleased me right from the start, because I enjoy dancing and I can't imagine a wedding reception being complete without a waltz.

Since Levin made no move to get to his feet, my father asked me to dance, which, by all the normal rules of etiquette, was quite acceptable. The best man and matron of honour, Dieter and Dorit, were next on to the dance-floor, followed by others. My father was a good dancer, which was news to me, and I was happy to have this chance to be fairly close to him in this uncomplicated way.

'You can't imagine what a relief it is to me,' he said, 'to see you well taken care of. In two years, I'll be retiring, and on my pension I'll no longer be in a position to help you out.'

'Father, I've been holding down a job of my own for the past six years!'

He nodded, vaguely. By this time, we were in the middle of a tango, when I suddenly caught sight of Levin close by.

For a strict non-dancer, he was getting on all too well, and Margot, who was becoming commoner by the minute, was putting on an erotic performance. My enjoyment was gone in a flash.

After the last tango, I went and sat with my boss. She had shot me a pleading glance, desperate for help. The good Dr Schneider had had a few too many. Although his wife, rather older than him, was seated only a few places away, he was pestering my boss with ambiguous compliments. Naturally, she was perfectly able to handle this sort of thing. All the same, I felt obliged to come to her aid. 'My parents would love to meet you,' I said, and she was only too glad to get to her feet and change places.

Dr Schneider was peering at me intently. 'Yes, young Levin's got his hands on a good thing all right,' he said. Then he went on at great length about his friendship with old Graber and how closely and loyally he had been connected with his whole family for decades. 'I'm looking forward to you moving to Viernheim and hope I'll soon be able to treat the fourth generation.'

'No way,' I thought. 'In the event I do have a child, I'll certainly not be taking it anywhere near this old fossil's surgery!' But of course I kept up the charm.

'He was a tough old fellow, my friend Hermann,' the doctor went on. 'Hard as nails. Had to be, or he'd never have got anywhere. He came from a very modest background, you know. His son was the complete opposite, but it's obvious now that Levin, too, knows exactly what he wants for himself. Ah yes, he's gone now, Hermann is, and yet he could well have enjoyed a long and happy old age. A death like that I wouldn't wish on my worst enemy.'

My heart stopped. But hadn't Levin told me that it had been all over in a flash? 'Hunky-dory', he had said!

'What do you mean?' I asked, my voice flat. 'I thought he had died, quite peacefully, over breakfast.'

'I wasn't there when it happened. But it was clear right away that he had suffered excruciating spasms, you could see it on his distorted features and his tightly clenched hands; he had obviously been trying to call for help right to the last –

72

the telephone was lying on the floor, the tablecloth had been dragged off. Not every death from a bad heart is quick and peaceful.'

These words were like hammer-blows. Up till then, I had been able to suppress the part I played in Hermann Graber's demise, consoling myself with the thought that he would have died soon anyway.

The doctor could see I wasn't feeling well. But he took it to be the usual bride's anxiety. 'Go outside and get a breath of fresh air,' he advised.

Ever since I had been living close to Schwetzingen Castle, I had loved the park as if it were my very own. I would often sit in the open-air theatre, reading; I would find a spot next to the artificial ruins and have a picnic, sit meditating in the mosque or settle on a bench on the lakeside and feed the ducks. On my wedding day, I would have loved to be able to enjoy this garden hand in hand with Levin, but now instead I was standing all on my own in front of that stone sphinx, and like all sphinxes, it was giving me its cat-like smile and saying nothing. It wasn't it that restored my composure, but the ancient trees, the birds, maybe even the gormless goldfish in the water. Within ten minutes I had myself firmly under control again. Now I was called Hella Moormann-Graber and had to reckon with being addressed as Frau Graber, which would be an eternal reminder of old Hermann. I would have to get used to it.

I made up my mind to return to the company of the wedding guests as quietly and unobtrusively as I could, to mingle with the happy crowd and join in the dancing. I avoided the broad, arrow-straight paths and instead sneaked along behind the trees and the boxwood shrubs sculpted into spheres, heading for the ballroom. The park was far from deserted; as well as some late-season tourists, a number of our guests were also wandering about, cooling off after the feasting and dancing. I was about to pass that particular bench that was just made for loving couples, on which I had often sat myself. It was occupied. I paused behind some bushes, convinced I had heard something which made my blood freeze. I was right. Margot was sitting there. But no, not with Dieter – the man beside her was Levin.

For the second time, my stomach turned over. The two of them were engaged in animated conversation. They were sitting close together, talking intimately.

'Well, yes,' Levin was saying, 'she does look like a little wire-haired terrier, you're right, but she does everything I want, and that's something you can't always expect of a terrier.'

So that cat on heat had the temerity to compare me with a terrier? I had the urge to rush out and bite her.

'C'mon, Levin, I'm freezin' 'ere!' said Margot, and the two of them got to their feet. I followed without them noticing.

The dancing was still in full swing in the ballroom. I had hardly merged back into the throng when Dieter took me by the arm. 'I've missed you,' he said, politely. 'This dance is mine.'

Thank heavens it wasn't Levin who spoke these words – I wouldn't have been able to control myself. To Dieter's amazement, I snuggled close to him, as if he were the bridegroom. He hardly reacted; it was only his good manners that prevented him from shaking me loose. But after two dances (for I made no move to let go of him) we had struck up an understanding in gliding around the floor that seemed to give him pleasure.

Margot was dancing as if in ecstasy with my brother (whose wife's face was pure vinegar), and Levin with Dorit. He gave me a wave, playing the innocent. I was by now fully in command of my expression and flashed back a charming smile. It had no doubt at last occurred to Levin that it was his damned duty to dance with his newly-wed wife, and, when the next waltz came along, it was my turn.

Levin was a good head taller than me, and I'm sure we didn't look like a dream couple. But I at least tried to act as if we were and to look radiant. Everyone, and especially my narrow-minded parents, was watching us, very touched. All sorts of bloody fairy-tale themes came to my mind to the three-four beat, not least Bluebeard's last wife, who stumbled across the dismembered corpses of her predecessors. In a way,

I had gone crazy, split into two persons, the blonde bride who, envied by everyone, celebrates the happiest day of her life, and the shaggy terrier who, without so much as thinking, tears a cat to shreds, not to mention the odd stray item of big game.

On my wedding evening, the only person who kissed me was Dorit. When, at last, I lay in bed beside Levin, we were both dead beat, so exhausted that we fell asleep at once. He had had a lot to drink, I had blisters on my feet.

'With new shoes, you've got to walk them in first,' remarked Frau Hirte.

The next day, my parents wanted to view our future home before they drove off again. While Margot knew very well that we could be expected around twelve, that didn't stop her still being in bed. In the meantime, she hadn't done so much as air the house, but had instead spread herself about the place; it was no longer the case that she occupied only the one floor. The tradesmen had yet to make a start on their renovation work, but they had put up scaffolding around the building, delivered the roof tiles and dumped the new baths and bathroom tiles. The house hardly presented a favourable picture; when Margot finally emerged in her faded pink housecoat, once again looking very much like a flea-bitten teddy bear, I was, on the one hand, relieved – looking like that she could hardly appeal to Levin – yet on the other, I felt let down in front of my family.

But my parents were far less interested in Margot than in the generous, upper-class layout of the villa; above all, they were entranced by the garden, with its tall pine trees which, with their kitschy German gloominess, were what appealed to me least. I had already considered having them felled and replaced by cherry and apple trees. The pampas grass in the front garden, too, went against my grain, but then again, Levin liked it, because, as a child, he had got up to all sorts of pranks with its tall spikes.

When at last my parents, and Bob too, had driven off, I

immediately brought up the subject of Hermann Graber's death. Levin played stupid.

'The old quack just wants a place in the limelight,' he said. 'I mean, I did see my own dead Grandpa myself, a picture of perfect peace, honestly. Are you going to believe that old blether rather than me?'

I nearly said 'Yes'. But was our marriage to start off with a row? And then there was also the business with Margot, though the last thing I wanted to hear was accusations of groundless jealousy.

I was not in the best of moods, and I regretted having taken a week's holiday from work. I would have loved to go off for a few days in Venice, but Levin shuddered at the prospect of doing the rounds of the sights of a city swamped by Yanks and Japs. He wanted to go to Hong Kong. We finally compromised, deciding to fly, when we next had holiday time, to East Asia, but to stay put at home for the moment.

I was almost glad when the time came for me to go back to work. True, Levin was very nice and made me presents of expensive-looking things I didn't really want, but deep down I knew that these were attempts at bribery. He hadn't married me just for my beautiful brown eyes.

'And what about you?' Frau Hirte put her oar in. This time, she hadn't fallen asleep for an instant.

'What do you mean, me?'

'What I mean is, you only took him because you wanted to have a child at last.'

'Well, so what if I did?' I said grumpily.

And now she was even coming at me with a quotation from the Bible: 'Suffer the little children to come unto me, and forbid them not: for of such . . .'

'Good night!' I said.

8

No doubt Frau Hirte rummages about in the drawer of my bedside table just as freely as I do in hers; all the same, I wouldn't like to think of her coming across Levin's postcards or Pavel's letters. Recently, I came up with a good haul: inside one of her many detective novels lay a photo. It shows her, dressed in a sporty kind of parka and pushing a man along in a wheelchair; apparently she gets her kicks by doing good works on the charity circuit. The cripple might well have been a good-looking man at one time, the model of a young revolutionary of the 1968 vintage, getting on a bit now, but with only a minimal shred of personality left recognizable.

Of late, she has been showing rather more interest in me, which, however, does not stretch to the extent of her telling me anything about herself; there's probably not much worth talking about anyway. In any case, it's nothing short of ridiculously boring when she natters on with her Frau Römer about dogs, doctors and former colleagues. Maybe that explains why she never tires of urging me to get on with my story.

Levin never came straight out with it, but he obviously expected me to sign the fortune over to him; all sorts of casual remarks and tokens of affection were his way of keeping the idea in my mind. I took advantage of one such situation to raise once again the question of why Dieter and Margot had got married.

'She once provided him with an alibi,' said Levin, after some hesitation.

'A false alibi, then?'

'What else?'

After a good deal more probing, I learned that Margot had been pregnant at the time.

'By Dieter?'

'Probably.'

And what had become of the child?

'Margot was taking drugs, even during the pregnancy, the kid arrived far too prematurely and died.'

That distressed me so much that he was hardly able to calm me down again.

'It had its good side, too,' Levin said. 'It gave Margot such a scare she stopped fixing.'

While I did feel slightly sorry for Margot, I still couldn't come to terms with her irresponsibility. And what was the business with the alibi? There, he was giving nothing away.

At this time we were driving out to Viernheim every weekend to inspect the builders' progress. By now, I had already developed a passionate attachment to my house. A conservatory had always been one of my dreams. It was built on as an extension to the rear of the house and afforded a wonderful view out on to my spacious garden. In my mind's eye, I could see a profusion of flowers and plants for every season of the year, rattan furniture with Indian silk cushions just inviting you to linger, a parrot swinging gently back and forth among tropical lianas. This was to be my own paradise.

What I didn't in the least like was the fact that Dieter and Margot were making no signs of a move to pack their things. Levin reckoned that, since we were not planning on moving in until after the renovation work was finished anyway, it would be no trouble to let them have two rooms for themselves in the meantime, especially since they hadn't found anything suitable yet.

'They're not even looking around for a flat,' I said.

'Of course they're looking,' Levin protested. 'But you know yourself the state the property market's in. You don't just find something overnight.'

Dieter had obviously been given some kind of pay-off, I had no idea how much, for what else could he be living off? Margot, too, appeared to be drawing her wages as before, which did make some sense, since after all she was there to open up for the workers, sweep up the mess behind them and ply them with something to drink.

I considered two bathrooms to be necessary – up till then the house had had only one – for our children should have the freedom to splash around in their own one, but did we need two kitchens as well?

'If we're hard up at any time,' said Levin, 'we can always let one floor, and a kitchen makes each level into a complete flat.'

'If it really comes to it and we're stuck, we can always get a conversion done,' I decided and would listen to no further argument.

When, after three months' building work, we finally moved in, Dieter and Margot were still living there, and we had to share the kitchen. The seeds of disaster were already sown.

I am tidy, almost perfectionist by nature, otherwise I could never have become a pharmacist. Even as a little girl, I loved baking cakes and biscuits, weighing out everything precisely to the last gram on the letter scales. My kitchen sparkles, everything there is exactly according to a system, I can lay my hand on everything I need with my eyes shut. Levin's sloppiness was enough to irritate me, but I would forgive him, the way one forgives a child.

My kitchen is a miniature laboratory, my empire of spices, aromas and experiments, in which I pick myself up after a long hard day behind the shop counter. From my grandmother, I have an ancient doll's shop with thirty wooden drawers delicately decorated with little porcelain nameplates, and I keep my herbs and spices in these.

That was my first shock. Vanilla, cinnamon, cloves and cardamom were no longer kept separate in their own dainty little drawers, but all crammed together into a shocking pink plastic container for cheap coffee. And instead of them, Margot had dumped sticking plasters, rubber bands, freezer labels, paperclips, an eraser and similar non-food ware in my miniature drawers. I nearly had a fit. I gathered these disgusting articles together and flung them into Margot's refuse tip of a bedroom. She got the message all right: war had been declared.

As a result of the move, my life had become somewhat more complicated. My first flat had been a stone's throw from the chemist's, from Schwetzingen it was a fair bit further, but now I had half an hour's drive to work. Still, for the time being at least, I was unwilling to sacrifice my career and my independence. So I was always the first to leave in the mornings.

Levin should have been the next one out of the house, to get to the university, but I had a sneaking suspicion that he was no longer pursuing his studies seriously and preferred to catch up on his sleep. Probably only once I already had a few hours' work behind me would breakfast be taken in my villa. The thought of them all together at table constantly conjured up an unpleasant picture for me.

It had to be said in Dieter's favour that he was by no means idle; immediately after his release from prison, he had applied for jobs, but he had found nothing in the profession in which he was qualified, selling insurance. One haulage firm, where he had also applied, offered him a temporary post as a relief driver. While driving a lorry, which he had learnt during his military service, hardly matched up to the level of his qualifications, he had accepted.

From then on, Dieter was frequently out on the road; it wasn't a job with solid long-term prospects or regular hours, but I gave him full credit for not considering it beneath his dignity. On his days off, he worked in the garden, he papered and painted the two rooms he and Margot lived in, as well as doing other useful jobs around the house. Levin had passed Hermann Graber's Mercedes on to him.

Whenever Dieter and Margot were together, I didn't let the pair of them out of my sight. How did they get on with each other? It was difficult to say exactly; there existed a certain camaraderie, a sense of sharing the same destiny, but, as far as I could make out, neither sexual tension nor tenderness. Were they sleeping together? Since they were both young and shared Hermann Graber's double bed, then one could only suppose they did.

Levin and I lived in four rooms on the ground floor. In Levin's 'study den' there was a second television set, always on. It was my plan to move our bedroom and, naturally, the children's rooms, to the first floor later on. In the basement was what had been Margot's room, while up under the roof there were two attic rooms which had originally been set aside for the domestic staff. That was where all those items of old man Graber's furniture, which neither we nor the other couple could put to any use, were piled up. Of course, Levin was right; my house was much too large for two people.

Which was why, as someone always with a social conscience, I didn't find it easy when I tried to give Dieter and Margot formal notice to quit.

Nor could they appreciate what I was getting at. 'Are we being a nuisance?' asked Dieter in consternation.

I would have loved to be able to answer that he was no bother to me at all, but his slovenly wife most certainly was. I was embarrassed – what sort of reasons could I come up with? Obviously Levin, despite all his claims to the contrary, had never once told them they would have to look for other accommodation.

But she was constantly working, Margot insisted, offended and obsequious at one and the same time. And Margot really was doing her bit, but everything she did filled me with revulsion. She washed down the many wooden staircases with dirty water and had obviously never even heard of such a thing as floor polish. Everything in the upstairs rooms stank, and this fustiness followed me to every corner of the house. Apparently Margot never opened a window in their bedroom, and she certainly didn't in the kitchen. I couldn't bring myself to touch the wiping-up cloth she used; I had one of my own, which I tried to keep hidden from her. But she soon tracked it down and made it so grubby and horrible that I came home almost every day with a newly purchased stock of cloths. Another thorn in my flesh was the fact that she always addressed Levin saucily as 'Clever-clogs'.

I detested her in a very physical way and never wanted to let anything she had cooked pass my lips. In the evenings, I would stand at the stove, which I could never get really clean, concocting an elegant meal for Levin and myself, but more and more I would be nauseated by the state of the refrigerator, with all the cheap margarine, rancid soft cheese – always lying unwrapped – and mouldy sausage that Margot stored in it. One day, Levin asked, 'Are you pregnant, or what? You've become so pernickety about food.'

Unfortunately, I didn't get pregnant as quickly as that, but all the same I knew there was no point in obsessively waiting for it. Did Levin's question suggest that he was anticipating it, too? That's the way I interpreted it.

Once the conservatory was finished, I felt a new surge of *joie de vivre*. I went mad buying plants – a van crammed full of them drove up in front of the house. Now I could sit the whole year round surrounded by greenery and gaze out into the garden at mealtimes, I could even sway gently in a hammock with a book, dream dreams and shut out the musty fug in the house, because out here there was always a slight aroma of moist vegetation. Every day, I looked forward to getting home to water my plants, to give Tamerlane a little push in the hammock and then to eat out here and not in my sadly desecrated kitchen.

'Now that everything's finished,' I suggested one day in high spirits, 'we should maybe throw a little house-warming party. Dorit and Gero haven't even been here yet, and my boss is bursting with curiosity . . .'

Levin was all for it. My one problem was Margot. Here at home, she loafed about most of the time in an unkempt state (in a tiger-striped mini-skirt and green plush slippers), but the moment there was any prospect of a special occasion, that brought the certainty of her metamorphosis into the bird of paradise of the party, and I found that even more repellent than the smell of boiled cabbage around the house.

But could she be excluded? A helping hand with washing glasses and clearing up was not to be sneezed at – at least, that was Levin's argument. I would have been only too happy to clear up on my own.

In general, I had to be careful not to give all too clear

expression to my aversion to Margot, for Levin had absolutely no sympathy with it. He didn't see the sausage in the fridge as mouldy, found the cooker was clean enough and reckoned I should consider myself lucky to have a helping hand around the house since my work seemed to be putting me under some strain.

Autumn was coming, and it was getting dark early. Two weeks before the big party, I was on night duty. While I had nodded off, a window in the back shop was smashed, a junkie on the hunt for supplies. Still half asleep, I confronted him, the alarm system went off, so the crazed idiot took a swing at me and I fell to the floor. The police were on the spot very promptly, managed to nab the thief a couple of streets away and then set about assessing the extent of the damage.

My boss was phoned and she came rushing on the scene and packed me off home in the end. Apart from a cut head, which she attended to herself, I had suffered nothing more than a slight shock. The police offered to drive me home, although when they heard that I lived in Viernheim, they seemed relieved that I declined their offer.

In the evenings, I usually drove my car straight into the garage, but that night I just hadn't the strength left. I crept quietly across the gravel path up to the front door. Everybody seemed to be asleep, but then it was three in the morning after all. Suddenly, I saw a beam of light shining on the back lawn, obviously coming from the conservatory. With a stab of fear, I put my front door key away again and felt my way carefully round to the back of the house. Were burglars at work here, too?

In the conservatory there were neither burglars nor forced doors to be seen. With a weird expression on his face, Levin was lying in the hammock. To my dismay, he was naked, with only the cat lying like a fig-leaf on his lower abdomen. What was he staring at so intently?

I had to move round to another corner of the garden to be able to get a sight of what his eyes were glued on. Margot was dressed in nothing but a black suspender belt and red boots, and she had perched her purple knickers coquettishly on her head. There was a peep-show going on in my conservatory while I was assumed to be at work. But where was Dieter?

I stood watching far too long. Suddenly it was clear to me where Margot's talents lay. She was displaying herself to Levin in a way that I considered perverted and disgusting, and was doing things I would never in my life have had anything to do with. I only slipped away when Levin handed her a small envelope and slumped back, exhausted, in my hammock, because the unappetizing coupling had reached its conclusion.

I went back through the garden to the front door, opened it and crept into the bedroom. Mechanically, I undressed, cleaned my teeth, rubbed cream into my face and went to bed. I was shivering so much my teeth were chattering. The bed next to me remained unoccupied.

I couldn't sleep, nor could I cry. I was in no state to dispel my ferocious rage and misery by counting sheep. Over and over again, I pictured the scene. In fact, I had never suffered from a sexual inferiority complex, I had always enjoyed physical love, as, for the most part, had my partners. Where Levin was concerned, things had been slightly different; for a young, healthy man, he had, to put it diplomatically, never really performed to adequate capacity. Obviously he required more powerful stimulation than my tender caresses and gentle snuggling.

What Margot had presented there was all too much of a routine. No doubt she was a professional who had in earlier days made a living on the streets and working in strip clubs and peep-shows. For all that, she had looked like some mindless robot, programmed by a higher power. True, she wasn't fixing regularly any more, but there could be no doubt he had given her some kind of drug as her reward.

In a peculiar way, these thoughts calmed me down a little; Levin's actions could be seen in the same light as if he had, like, say, his grandfather before him, been visiting a brothel. But then my conservatory was not a brothel! I was not long married to Levin, and Margot was his friend's wife. What it amounted to was that she had, by this act of depravity, soiled and polluted my conservatory just as she had my kitchen.

I'll have everything disinfected, I thought, Levin will have to move out and he won't get a penny out of the divorce.

Towards morning, I had to go to the toilet. I couldn't stop myself, but crept into the living room and from there took a peek into the conservatory. Levin was sleeping the sleep of the dead in the hammock – under my Irish woollen blanket. An old saw came to my mind: 'He who sleeps commits no sin, he who has sinned will sleep the better for it'.

Frau Hirte let out an evil chortle.

Levin would not be expecting me home until the next afternoon, since normally, after night duty, I would have had to stay on at the chemist's all the following day. Had Margot sneaked into bed beside her husband after it was over? Was Dieter here at all? Were there always such orgies going on whenever I was out of the house? Did Margot's recent black eye have anything to do with Dieter's discovery of what was going on?

And Margot's dead child: was Levin its father? I was shuddering with cold and nausea. Still trembling, I went into the kitchen to make a cup of camomile tea. Propped against the kitchen cupboard, I waited for the water to boil. Slowly, the door, which had been ajar, swung open, and my tom-cat Tamerlane crept silently in. With his tail stiffly erect, he rubbed against my legs and demanded attention. Just what, I wondered, would the animal have told me if it could speak?

As I drank my tea, I decided to act for the time being as if nothing had happened. But it wasn't Levin who followed Tamerlane into the kitchen. It was Dieter.

9

Pavel couldn't always leave the children at Dorit's, so it wasn't long before he brought them with him to the hospital again. It was obvious that, in those circumstances, he would not be able to wait long.

'Have you any more dolly-cheese for me?' asked Lene.

It was the jam that Kolya was keen on. 'But we don't like the burny sausage, Hella, you can keep it for yourself,' he said.

All the same, Pavel packed the meat paste with the peppercorns away with the rest. 'We'll take it to Alma.'

Once we were on our own again, Frau Hirte, with unexpected curiosity, asked, 'Who is Alma?'

'Pavel's wife.'

'You've lost me completely now.'

'All will be revealed, Frau Hirte.'

'Just one more question: Where is Alma now?'

'In the loony bin.'

Her eyes went wide, and I got a kick from her bewilderment.

'I'm itching to know what happens next with Margot,' she said. 'I could never have summoned up as much patience as you did.'

'Next instalment, eight o'clock,' I promised.

Dieter was taken aback to find me in the kitchen.

'Don't you have night duty?' he asked.

Falteringly, I told him the story of the break-in, and he expressed his regrets.

'It seems to have knocked you back a fair bit,' he said, pouring the water into the teapot. Unaccustomed as I was to such little favours, I burst into tears at his concern. Dieter took me in his arms like an ailing child. Tamerlane was consumed with jealousy and tried to push his way between us.

Like myself, Dieter sometimes had to get up early to go to work. He drank a cup of tea standing up. In the end, I inquired, as innocently as I could manage, where Levin had got to.

Dieter was puzzled. The last he had seen of him, he said, was at supper, and Levin hadn't said anything about going out. 'Maybe he's hanging in the hammock,' he said, jokingly. 'That is his favourite place, isn't it? I'll go and have a look.'

'If he is there, don't wake him,' I begged.

The cat shot off after him. With a look of complete bafflement on his face, Dieter came back. 'The crazy bugger's dossing in the conservatory,' he said and left, after urging me to get myself straight back off to bed.

It was midday before there was a sound of movement in the house, then I heard the toilet flushing. Suddenly, Levin was standing by our bed, looking at me, disconcerted. Once again I went through my story about the junkie and showed him my wound.

'When did you get home?' This was all that interested him.

'I don't know.'

There were signs of anxiety in Levin's face as he searched my long-suffering expression for traces of reproach. 'I must have dropped off in the conservatory,' he said. 'Did you come looking for me?'

'I took a strong sleeping pill and tumbled straight into bed.'

Apparently, my bandage reassured Levin a little, but he seemed bothered that I hadn't got in touch with him after such a shock. 'Why didn't you phone from Heidelberg?' he said. 'I'd have come and picked you up.'

'Oh, for goodness sake,' I said, 'that would have taken twice as long. And anyway, I didn't want to leave the car there. But now, just let me sleep a bit longer.'

Levin left me, and I got back to my brooding. Was I going to have to take him to task? Revenge? Divorce? I couldn't come to any clear decision. Was it absolutely necessary to act hastily and in doing so destroy something that couldn't be put together again?

*   *   *

When pangs of hunger forced me to get up during the afternoon, Levin bustled about and made some toast for me. At least his conscience is bothering him, I thought. But not as badly as all that, it seemed, for once he had heard that I was feeling better, he raced off in the Porsche.

I was still sitting in the kitchen in my dressing-gown when Margot came in. No doubt she was acting under instructions, for right away she asked if there was anything she could do for me.

'You bet,' I said.

From that moment on, I started giving Margot a rough time of it. Up till then, I had avoided giving her direct orders. Now and then I would mutter something about the cutlery needing polishing, or something of the sort, without looking straight at Margot. And sometimes she had taken note of such hints. Now I said, in no uncertain terms, that the refrigerator was to be washed out with water and vinegar, the oven had to be thoroughly cleaned, the bathtub and the toilet bowl, for all that they were new, were furred up, the pavement had to be swept and the fallen leaves in the drive had to be cleared up and put on the compost heap.

'We're not paying you to sit around doing absolutely nothing,' I said.

Margot flushed fiery red. She had always dusted and cleared up, she insisted.

'But how!' I snapped back, and she wasn't to forget that she was living here rent-free.

Levin had always been quite satisfied, she defended herself.

What did a man know about things like that, I snorted at her, and anyway, this was my house, not his.

Margot gaped at me. 'Hella, the house was Levin's grandad's,' she tried to put me right.

Without a word, I dug the will out of the desk drawer and spread it out under her nose.

She took a good look at it and then, shaking her head, said, 'That ain't right.'

A day or so later, when I was going out to the garage in the morning, I gave the big wicker basket a hefty kick, so that it tipped over and all the withered leaves from the magnolia swirled through the air again. The sight of them flying around gave me great satisfaction, and I thought, 'Some flowers for you, Margot.' At that moment, I noticed Dieter, who must have been following right behind me. Highly amused, he said, 'That's the way to work off your aggression! I'll sweep it all up again later.'

Rather embarrassed, I assured him I'd see to it. But in my rear-view mirror I could see that he didn't get into the Mercedes, but went to fetch a rake and a broom.

In the normal run of things, I saw Dieter only seldom. Whenever we did happen to meet, we'd exchange smiles. I once caught myself rather provoking one of these chance meetings. Did he perhaps quite like me, too? Once, he had left a book in the conservatory, with a note inscribed 'For Hella' beside it. Was it a present, or only on loan? It was a science-fiction novel, all about some scientist's utopian dreams. I was touched by that, because, unlike this gift, all Levin's presents only served his own preferences.

After my nocturnal discovery, I no longer fancied sleeping with Levin. But he hardly seemed to notice, for I had always been the one to take the initiative anyway, and so I was spared the awkward situation of having to reject his advances. Sooner or later, I thought, it's bound to dawn on him that the interval was longer than usual. But obviously he wasn't having to go without.

I wondered whether Dieter knew. Was he in fact nothing more than Margot's pimp? I didn't want to think ill of him. Yes, sure, he had gone off the straight and narrow once upon a time, but he was by no means a worthless sort. On the contrary, there was something chivalrous and reserved about him that I liked a lot.

Our party invitations had all been sent out well before those events threw everything into total confusion, and it was far too late for me to call off the whole thing. On the Friday before our do, I had taken the day off, and the first thing I did was to drive to the finest grocery stores in town. Soon, my car was filled with the most delicious smell of basil.

Then I disappeared for the rest of the day into the kitchen. Levin had driven off to the Palatinate to buy in supplies of wine – or, to be more exact, I had sent him off there. I kept Margot on the hop with menial tasks.

Suddenly, the doorbell was ringing like fury and Dorit burst in in her bustling, purposeful way. When we were students together, we had been, to all outward appearances, a pair of complete opposites, yet inseparable; I'm small, blonde and wiry, she is tall and slim with a beautifully groomed mane of black hair.

It did me good to park myself in the kitchen and have a good chinwag with Dorit while I peeled the vegetables. 'You don't exactly look like a happy newlywed,' she said straight off.

I put all the blame on Margot. 'I just can't bear living under the same roof as that woman,' I said. 'What do you think of her? I mean, you did meet her at the wedding.'

'I found her dreadful, common and vulgar, man-mad and stupid with it,' said Dorit. 'But her husband seemed not a bad sort.'

That was grist to my mill. 'Can you understand a man like that being married to such a horror?' I asked Dorit.

She gave her loud, husky alto laugh. 'Come on, Hella, you see these things day and daily. Of all the married couples I know, I prefer the one partner or the other. You always wonder what they see in each other. But one thing I do know, sometimes these marriages work quite well, even if no one can figure out how.'

Was Dieter and Margot's marriage working? Was it anything more than just a partnership on paper? 'Dorit, what advice would you give me: how can I get that damned bitch off my back?'

She thought for a while. 'Hard to say. You've probably no chance unless Levin plays along. He would have to be one hundred per cent behind you in a thing like this. But there you are, men are like that, all pals right down the line. But have you no good news to tell me?'

'You know very well you'd be the first to hear, but for the time being, no, I'm not pregnant yet,' I said sullenly.

Dorit gave me a hug. 'It'll come, you just have to be a bit patient. Is that why you're so depressed?'

I shook my head, and for a while we topped and tailed runner beans in silence.

With the life of abstinence we were leading at the moment, I was certainly not going to get pregnant, and that probably made much better sense than tying myself to such a Lothario.

Dorit could read at least part of my thoughts. 'Even at the wedding reception, you were cheesed off at Margot because she was going around throwing herself at all the blokes, but most of all at the great Levin – am I right?'

I didn't answer. In some respects, Dorit was my alter ego, she had studied pharmacy as well, and she was therefore every bit as fussy about strict cleanliness as I was, and she, too, was well versed in the alchemy of the kitchen, with a passion for little bottles, tins and drawers. But there was one thing where we were never of one mind, and that was my men-friends. Dorit had a really good husband, whose patent faithfulness (exactly what you'd expect of a man of his age) she would sometimes call into question just for a joke. What she did freely admit was that he was a respectable, presentable partner who was pulling down a good salary. The kind of characters I had collected about me up till then had quite simply filled her with revulsion.

My silence seemed to be an admission that she was right. She was certainly on the right track. 'You know, Hella,' she started again, 'I read somewhere recently, "Sexuality is power, and power, by its nature, is aggressive." Nicely put, wouldn't you say?'

'And what are we to draw from that?' I asked with some sarcasm.

'There's more,' said Dorit. 'Goodwill, dependability, loyalty and morality don't stand a chance when sex is involved – nature is much stronger than all our humanist and Christian commandments put together.'

'So am I supposed to be cheered by your philosophy?'

'Far from it,' she said. 'You've got to analyse this Margot. She has power over Levin, and, it would appear, over you too, for you're getting far too worked up over the silly trollop. If she can't behave properly, then simply kick her out!'

Naturally, there weren't so many guests at our housewarming as at the wedding – no relatives, no dignitaries or notables. Mind you, my boss was very welcome, because I really liked her. She brought along a shy grass widower called Pavel Siebert, a regular customer in her chemist's shop.

I was on the go right up to the last minute, cooking, clearing up, polishing glasses. When the first guest rang the doorbell, I was just doing a quick change in no time flat. I had bought myself a new dress – well, after all, I was supposed to be comfortably off, or, to be more accurate, rich. So I put on silk and cashmere, great-grandmother's six-stranded garnet necklace and Italian shoes with very high heels, so as to seem a little taller. I found teetering around on stilettos a bit strange at first, since, despite my lack of height, I had never owned anything but flat, sensible shoes.

As a matter of fact, I thought my husband might have remarked on my new appearance, but he didn't. He welcomed guests, poured out glasses of champagne and chatted, while Dorit and I accepted the flowers they brought and arranged them in vases.

Margot made her big entrance only once everyone had already arrived. I was fully expecting to see her in the same black creation with which she had soured my wedding. But no; she was wearing a bra-top in gold, a dog-collar necklace and tight black leather pants, with, at the rear, just at cheek height, holes punched in the leather. She fully achieved what she was aiming at: everyone fell immediately silent, staring at this picture either in consternation or with barely suppressed lust. I looked around for Dieter and finally spied him right in the background, leaning against the wall. His expression as he watched the reactions of the company was inscrutable. Pavel Siebert, too, had retreated into a corner, where he was engrossed in one of my grandfather's old dispensing notebooks.

Dorit pushed her way through to me. 'Gero thinks she's quite awful, so he says, but just look at him, eyes like organ-stops!'

I was well aware that friends and husbands of my girl-friends were passing whispered comments about Margot, but goggling with their eyes on stalks, just like Gero, and one or two were even poking their finger tips into the punched out holes. Levin was going about beaming with proprietorial pride. I felt like giving his face a good slap in front of the whole company. Even my boss had sized up the situation. Glass in hand, she came over to join Dorit and me. 'She's stealing the show from us, isn't she?' she commented. 'Hella, I'd dearly love to see round the house. The conservatory is a delight . . .'

I couldn't show her round the whole house, so I restricted myself to my own rooms. But I did manage to arrange it so that I told my boss, with Margot within earshot, 'The upstairs flat is going to be renovated within the next month, and that's where the bedrooms, guest rooms and nursery are to be.'

'You're right, Hella,' said my boss, 'to be planning for a nursery in good time. I missed out on that.'

My boss was divorced and childless, but nevertheless, thanks to the horse she owned, she always gave the impression of being a thoroughly contented woman.

To my great satisfaction, I noted that Margot had got the message. That she was offended was clear from her expression. 'Fine,' I thought, 'soon you'll be only too glad to leave of your own accord.'

Margot was not quite as stupid as Dorit and I liked to think. Whereas she would talk to us fellow members of the household without the slightest affectation, I was amazed to hear the different tones she put on – not without some effort – as she spoke to strange men. She was going on about all sorts of things, about local politics and the police (all a load of shit), about schools and cars (society gets what it deserves), and about the television programmes (again, not a good word to be said for them). None of the men was listening to what she was saying, but just ogling her cleavage.

I interrupted this idle prattling with a gruff order to get the glasses washed, and that right now. But, Margot protested, what about her good dress . . . ?

'You can hardly call that a dress,' I said, winning some laughs from the women present, who were very much on my side. 'And, while you're at it, you can put the quiche in the oven, heat it up for fifteen minutes and then serve it. But first, bring ten bottles of red wine up from the cellar.'

Margot passed this last job on to Levin, roped Dieter into the kitchen work and delegated the drying up to the very proper Gero.

Dorit saw this and couldn't help laughing. 'Hats off to her,' she said, 'I've never managed to get Gero to do that . . .'

After the quiche, which was eaten standing up, 'Porky' the butcher arrived about nine with a whole sucking pig which he sliced up on the kitchen table and divided into portions. I had prepared various salads, vegetables and potato gratin, set out little corners for people to sit and eat in the kitchen, the living room and the conservatory, and laid out crockery for self-service. Everything tasted fantastic, and I felt very pleased with myself.

Margot gave a hand at critical moments when everyone was looking for a place and a full plate, but no more than that. She had started flirting with 'Porky', a young assistant at the butcher's, and was keeping him back from his duties. With his big serving fork, he popped a huge piece of crackling, which he reckoned was the best part of the animal, into her mouth. I arrived on the scene just as Margot threw up, in a great spatter, all over the kitchen floor, causing the guests eating there to scatter, shrieking, and take flight from the room.

'I feel rotten,' groaned Margot and took to her heels.

And who else, apart from me, wiped the floor clean? Levin and Dieter gave me a cheery wave from a distance as I tried to gesture them to come and help. 'Right away, five minutes.'

In my silk dress, I knelt on the tiles to wipe up, the bitter stench making me feel sick myself. My disgust at Margot was taking on pathological proportions.

When everything was spotless once more, Dieter entered

the kitchen. 'So, what's up, Hella?' he said. 'Can I make myself useful in any way?'

Although he could not be expected to know what had happened, he bore the brunt of the full force of my fury. 'Get that bitch out of my house!' I bawled. 'She's puked all over my kitchen, and I've had to clear up the whole mess!'

In complete ignorance, Dieter asked why Margot hadn't done the cleaning up herself. By this time, Porky, whose trousers had caught part of it, and other refugees were filtering back into the kitchen to refill their plates, so I couldn't very well carry on making a scene with Dieter. But to this day, sucking pig with crispy crackling still makes my stomach heave.

10

'In my young days, I had a boyfriend who dumped me in a pretty lousy way,' said Frau Hirte, quite out of the blue.

Interesting.

'Actually, it was my own fault, I was far too gullible,' she went on.

'Well, you've just said you were young at the time . . .'

'That's no excuse. Can't you see that you, too, are making a crucial mistake?'

'Which one is that?'

'You have a completely wrong picture of reality.'

'Doesn't everybody?'

Frau Hirte shook her head.

If there's one thing I can't abide, it's old people who try to teach us a lesson, full of themselves and crowing about their experience of life and their knowledge of human nature. Up till now, she had never done this, but if this was to be the start of it, then I had spent my last night as her entertainer.

But she made no further move to pass judgement on me; her desire to know more got the upper hand. 'So how does the Margot story go on?'

Right, so this was the night I was going to make her blood run cold.

The day after our party, I was feeling wretched. A week early, and accompanied by unusually severe pains, my period arrived. Fortunately, it was a Sunday, so I decided to stay in bed. When the guests had finally left, late in the night, we hadn't bothered to clear up. So let the others get on with it.

Around midday, Levin shook me – almost gently by his standards – and said, 'A coffee wouldn't go wrong just now.'

I put on my suffering face. With a sigh, he made his own coffee and brought me a cup of tea, to put me in a good mood. 'There's a lot to be done,' he said. 'I'll go and get Margot and Dieter.'

Fine by me.

Feeling frail, I spent the day in my hidey-hole, pondering the situation. Nothing had gone the way I had planned. Though I had lots of money and my own house, a child, my most urgent desire, was nowhere in sight, nor, in the light of the absence of conjugal activity, was there any prospect of one. A husband I had, for sure, but a faithless, shallow and pretty idle one. When you came down to it, my one and only possibility was to break with him, fast, and find myself another; after all, I wasn't getting any younger. But how would my parents react? 'I knew it, right from the word go,' my mother would say. My father would go into a depression. Should I give it one more try with Levin? He was still young enough to have a greater sense of responsibility and a more serious attitude drummed into him. And when all is said and done, Hermann Graber had entrusted him to my care, so shouldn't I respect his last wishes? Anyway, I was feeling far too worn-out to come to any decision now.

I must have been brooding for a good couple of hours when there came an unexpected knock at my door. It was Dieter, to ask how I was getting on and was there anything I needed. 'We're just about finished, and everything's tip-top again,' he said. 'My head's thumping a bit. Do you fancy going for a walk?'

It would have done me more good to go out for an hour in the November mist than to lie in bed. Nevertheless, I declined the offer, the thought of Margot and Levin being left alone together in the house seemed unbearable, even though that would be the way it was again on Monday.

'Margot has to go!' I suddenly said out loud to myself.

97

Dismissal in writing, sent by registered post, was without doubt the first step. First thing tomorrow, I decided.

Thank heaven Margot did not put in an appearance at my bed of pain, but Levin came to ask whether I could do with another cup of tea or a packet-soup. 'Poor old Margot's not in the best of form either,' he remarked, quite inopportunely. I stared fixedly out of the window.

'Do you still have some holiday time to come this year?' he went on.

While I was in a foul mood, I was nevertheless curious.

Levin pulled a wedding announcement out of his pocket. A certain Dr Isabel Böttcher, BDS, was pleased to announce her forthcoming marriage to a colleague with a Spanish name a yard long. This, he said, was an old friend from his university days, who had fallen in love in Granada with a man from the best of families. A wedding in Andalusia – that, surely, was worth the jaunt, wasn't it?

For all that I was in a deep sulk, I wasn't averse to the idea. The celebrations were to take place the coming weekend. 'Do you think we'd still get a flight?' I asked.

Levin laughed. Flying was a bore, he said, and of course he'd be taking the Porsche.

I went back to suffering in silence. There was no way I could take any more than five days off, and going by car would be far too tiring. 'Go on your own,' I breathed.

Levin shook his head. 'On such a long stretch, you've got to change drivers now and then. Why don't you want to go? You're not as old as all that yet!'

It was meant as a joke, but it hurt me. 'Don't you have any idea what it means to have a job? I'm sure trips like that are the very thing for work-shy students.'

'That's okay by me,' said Levin. 'I'll just go and ask Dieter and Margot.'

'If you take Margot with you, I'm filing for divorce tomorrow.'

Levin looked at me warily. 'Jealous?'

'Of somebody like that? I can't stand her, and you know it. But I have no reason whatsoever to be jealous of her.'

Levin smelt trouble. He made off.

I learned that evening that he was aiming to start off at the crack of dawn, since Dieter couldn't go with him. 'So that you don't have to worry, I'll make a stop here and there on the way,' he said.

I took five valerian tablets, so as not to be about and have to make his coffee for him in the morning. Levin packed his things and probably slept a few hours beside me without my noticing he was there. When I awoke, both the Porsche and Levin were well on their way to Spain.

I took advantage of Levin's absence to do something underhand. I put an advert in the paper: FURNITURE FROM GRANDAD'S DAY TO BE DISPOSED OF CHEAP. Up till then we hadn't discussed the matter of whom Hermann Graber's gloomy sideboard and similar assets belonged to, to me or to him. The question was not touched upon in the will. Whether Levin was attached to the stuff or not, I wanted to clear the attic rooms and put them to good use, and my use at that. He had his little study, so where was mine?

Everything was sold in one afternoon. Now, I like beautiful old furniture very much, but that lot had never been beautiful, and I was glad to be rid of it. Dieter wasn't around, so he missed the spectacle of grasping characters with delivery vans, as well as genuine junk dealers and antiquarians, dragging the whole heap of garbage away, grunting and gasping. Margot stood there goggling, but she didn't give a second thought to whether what I had done was morally irreproachable or not. With a grin, she waved to a young couple who were loading up the black wardrobe with the carved capercaillies.

Over the weekend, I was alone with Margot, and I proposed to drive her like a slave. Several times, she asked what I wanted to do with the attics anyway. For visitors, for instance, I told her, or perhaps as a library or a hobby workroom.

These rooms up under the roof had not yet been renovated. A new fitted carpet would have to be laid, to go with some bright wallpaper. Margot groaned. It wouldn't be worth the effort of cleaning the place out first, she reckoned. In a way, she was right at that, but on principle I didn't want the worst of the dirt and the cobwebs in the house, they could give rise to vermin.

We scrubbed and swept together. 'I was right,' Margot remarked, trying to be matey, 'I always reckoned the little half-pint had the strength of an ox.'

It was meant as a compliment. I said nothing, but she went prattling on.

She was sure Levin would be on his road home by now, maybe even in Barcelona, because it was always great to get back to your own bed . . .

I felt my flesh creeping.

It cost me some effort, in that moment of almost intimate togetherness, to bring up the subject of her dismissal again. But when she kept on talking about 'our Levin', I couldn't restrain myself any more.

'It is of no interest to you whatsoever when my husband is coming back,' I exclaimed. 'The only thing that should be concerning you is finding somewhere else to live as soon as you can. If you're not going to do it of your own free will, I'll get a lawyer on to it. After all, as you no doubt know, there's no such thing as a rent contract between us.'

Margot resorted to servile pleading. She could move out of the first-floor flat and live up here with Dieter, then I would have four extra rooms, she said.

'How do you figure that?' I countered. 'Up here there's no bathroom and no kitchen, the water-pipes only come up to the first floor.'

Well, she suggested, looking like a frightened rabbit, we could get that done.

'Is that so? And who's going to pay for it? You, maybe?'

I had taken a particular fancy to the dormer windows in the attic. I could picture quite clearly my secret little refuge up here, my own little empire, with entry prohibited to everyone else living in the house. The windows were dulled by a thick layer of grime.

By this time, Margot had worked herself up into a frenzy of effort, fetching fresh water and smelly cloths from her own flat. Obviously, she felt she could get round me that way. In fact, the window frames were of indestructible quality, and needed no more than a fresh coat of paint. I sat on the windowsill and tried to get a hold of the shutters to swing them shut and assess how far they had rotted. They were solidly built, too, but of course the paint was flaking off. Margot set to work on the second window with a bucket of water.

'These shutters will have to be taken off their hinges, and Dieter'll have to strip them down and paint them,' I said.

Oh, he'd certainly do that, Margot assured me eagerly.

I climbed up on to the sill and tried to unhinge the shutter, but to no avail.

'That's too 'eavy for us, that's man's work,' said Margot disapprovingly. But I had got the bit between my teeth. 'Hold on to me, Margot,' I ordered.

Margot grabbed my legs and held me in a vice-like grip. I could smell her sweat. Unfortunately, I was too short in the arms to get a firm hold on the shutter. 'A drop of oil on the hinges,' I said, 'and then it'll be child's play.'

I ran downstairs to get my sewing-machine oil.

When I got back upstairs, Margot was kneeling on the windowsill. She was red in the face with effort. 'Hella, c'mon an' lift me up!' she said, all eagerness. 'I got longer arms 'n you!'

I stepped forward and reluctantly held her by the ankles. Her legs were red and blue mottled, and a dark stubble was sprouting after having recently been shaved. Her shabby leggings reached down no further than her knees. Out of her green slippers peeked corpse-yellow calloused heels. I was unspeakably repelled, but what really robbed me of all composure was a fine rivulet of sweat that was slowly and steadily dribbling down from her trouser leg towards my right hand.

She stood up from her crouching position. With a lurch, she suddenly caught hold of the shutter with both hands and, because of the unexpected weight of it, started to sway.

At that very instant, the greasy trickle of sweat reached me, and in a spontaneous reaction of indescribable disgust, I abruptly let go of her. Margot crashed down, still gripping the shutter with both hands. Horrified, I stared downwards. Two storeys below me, she lay there, dead or alive, I couldn't tell. In my haste, I knocked over the bucket of filthy water, tripped over the brush, staggered to my feet again and tore down the stairs as if pursued by the Furies.

It took me only seconds to get out into the garden where Margot lay on the stone flags of the terrace. She was still breathing, but unconscious. I felt her pulse, which was only just discernible. What was I to do? I was all alone in the house.

Naturally, I rang the emergency services. Two ambulance-men and an emergency doctor took Margot off to hospital. On the verge of fainting, I tried to call Dieter's haulage firm and babble out the words that they should contact him. There was only an answering machine running. Maybe Levin could be reached in Spain via the message service on the radio.

I phoned Dorit. In a toneless voice, I told her Margot had fallen out of the attic window.

'Is she dead?' asked Dorit in consternation.

'No, but they couldn't tell me yet how badly injured she is.'

'My God, you sound at the end of your tether,' said Dorit. 'You didn't see it happen, did you?'

'Not directly, but I was in the same room. Then I saw her lying down below. It was horrible.'

'How can anyone just fall out of a window?' asked the level-headed Dorit. 'That's the sort of thing that only happens to children . . .'

'She was trying to take the shutters off, because they needed painting.'

Dorit whistled through her teeth. 'Well, we shouldn't speak ill even of the badly injured, but it really is a piece of irresponsible nonsense to try to take on work like that on one's own!'

I made no effort to put her right.

'Everything will be fine,' she said, soothingly, 'and maybe she'll learn her lesson from this. Now you just calm down for a start. And if you feel like it, do come over here!'

I would have loved to drive to Heidelberg to let Dorit

mother me. But I was in no condition to drive a car, and I had to wait for Dieter.

In an effort to clear my head, I made myself some strong coffee, but I brought it all up again at once. Then I went back up the stairs and had a look at the scene of the crime. With binoculars, I did a sweep of all the houses that bordered on our garden at the back. Gero had friends who lived there too. Could anyone have observed anything from there? No, the pine trees I hated so much blocked the line of sight. Even with the binoculars, I couldn't have made out from my side whether anyone in those houses had been cleaning their windows. This fact calmed me a little. And anyway, neither neighbours nor passers-by had rushed up to stand and gape when the ambulance had driven up.

The problem was Margot herself. She knew I had let go of her. What could I come up with in mitigation? Revulsion was no excuse. What if I had been stung by a wasp? 'Nonsense,' I scolded myself out loud, there were no wasps about in November. Maybe a particularly nasty spider? That was possibly a little more plausible than a mere drop of sweat.

An hour later, I phoned the hospital. Was I a relative, they inquired. No, just an acquaintance. Then they couldn't give out any information, but it was vital that her next of kin be alerted right away and that they should come to the hospital. I promised to take care of that. Were Margot's parents alive? I didn't even know her maiden name. Whom should I ask? I phoned one of Levin's friends, but he couldn't help.

When Dieter got back at last, I ran towards him as he entered the drive. He could tell at once from my face that there was something wrong. 'I'll drive you to Margot, she's in hospital,' I stammered, pausing only to collect my coat. In the wardrobe mirror, I noticed I was still wearing the headscarf I had put on to do the dusting.

During the short trip, I told him the same story as I had given Dorit.

We were shown into the intensive care ward. Margot lay, in a deep coma, plugged into machines and tubes. A doctor led us outside, took Dieter with him and gave him an update on Margot's condition. As I learned later, she was beyond hope. Dieter was allowed to sit by her bed, while I waited outside. Two hours later, she was dead.

Dieter let me drive him back in mute silence. Once we were home, I led him into the kitchen and made him some tea and set a glass of brandy down beside it. He drank only the tea.

I hadn't a clue whether I should try to say something to comfort him, and if so, what. 'She can't have suffered,' I said. 'She lost consciousness at once.'

'Good God!' was all he could say. 'She's always had such a hard life. Here, in this house, at last things were going right for her, and that's it over already. She was as happy as Larry to have a nice home, thanks to your generosity, with a bathroom, a place that was heated . . .'

That was too much. I started howling and couldn't stop. Dieter stroked my hair. About his own emotions, he was stonily silent.

On the following Monday, I had to go back to work. Probably that was the best medicine. In the afternoon, Dieter phoned me at the chemist's, something he had never done. Levin hadn't got back yet, but the police had been there. In the case of accidents resulting in severe injuries or fatalities, investigations were a matter of routine. Since I was the sole witness, I was to call in at the police station in Viernheim directly after the shop closed.

I got a fright. 'What did they want to know?' I asked.

'What they were most interested in having a look at was the attic, the window and the height of the drop. They photographed the smashed shutter too, and the plush slippers.'

Admitting to having been in the same room had been a mistake. But when I described the situation to Dorit and Dieter, I had had to assume that Margot would survive and give her own version of the story. Then I would have brought the spider into play. Our two statements would not have been identical.

*   *   *

At the police station, I had to wait, and got myself into an increasingly worse state of anxiety. When they finally did take my statement, though, the whole thing no longer seemed quite so dramatic after all.

'Were you and Frau Krosmansky good friends?' I was asked.

I restrained myself. 'We lived in the same house . . .'

How did I get to know her, and when was that? Had there been no one else in the house? I didn't like these questions at all.

In the end, I had to accept a mild reproach from the police officer: it was a well-known fact that most serious accidents occurred in the home. How could anyone be so irresponsible as to clamber about in slippers on attic windowsills on a dull November Sunday and try to take down shutters?

'It all happened so quickly,' I said. 'We had this great urge to clear the decks in the attic rooms over the weekend, and to do it without the help of the menfolk. I was cleaning the right-hand window and wasn't really paying much attention to what Frau Krosmansky was doing. Suddenly, I heard this horrible shriek and when I looked, she was already lying down below.'

I had already reminded myself beforehand that my fingerprints, as well as Margot's, would be evident on both windows; there was no aspect of my statement that could be contradicted. I signed the statement and was about to get off home.

'One last question,' said the policeman when I was already at the door. 'How did the Krosmansky couple come to be living in Hermann Graber's house – I mean, your house – in the first place?'

'Well, they were acquaintances of my husband,' I said coolly.

The two policemen exchanged glances. 'Our good old Levin yet again,' said the older of the two meaningfully.

Dieter had very thoughtfully set the table, the kettle was whistling and a tempting aroma was coming from the oven.

The tea did me a lot of good.

'I suppose they told you both of us have a police record,' Dieter probed.

'Who do you mean by "both of us"?' I asked. He meant himself and Margot. But no, the police probably also had some kind of code of confidentiality, because they hadn't mentioned a word about the Krosmanskys' past lives.

'They'll be surprised at you living under the same roof as us,' Dieter went on.

I hadn't thought of that till now.

Dieter took a vegetable stew out of the oven, and I was happy not to be left alone with my thoughts.

11

*The night sister, who came to take our temperatures last thing
before changing shifts, looked with some concern at my sweat-soaked
nightdress. I wasn't feeling well. After showering, I put on one of
Dorit's pretty nightdresses.*

*I squinted over to Frau Hirte. Had she been listening during the
night or had she been asleep? How did she take Margot's death?*

*Positively, it seemed. When our eyes met, she said, 'A very good
morning to you!' and then, to my complete surprise, she rather
awkwardly suggested we should get on first-name terms. 'I'm called
Rosemarie,' she said, almost conspiratorially.*

*Later on, she asked, 'Is Levin still in the land of the living?' She
was no doubt expecting that, from now on in my story, people were
going to bite the dust, one after the other, just like the ten little
niggers.*

Levin wasn't back the next day either. Dieter had taken the
trouble to do some phoning around in Granada, since he
spoke a little Spanish. The young couple were away on their
honeymoon, he learned, and all the guests had left.

I was not in the least concerned about Levin, even if
Dieter thought I was. If anything really were to happen to
my husband, considering the way he drove, then I'd hear
about it soon enough. The peace and quiet without Levin
and Margot around was doing me good. I wanted to make
the most of this breathing space that fate had presented me
with. Dieter had a way of quietly turning up in the kitchen
every now and then, which pleased, rather than disturbed me.
The only worries I had centred around my cat, Tamerlane.
Since Margot's death, he would hardly eat a thing, he was in

mourning. While it had become obvious to me that he took advantage of my absences to snuggle down in the upstairs flat, I wouldn't have believed of him that he could have developed an affection for my enemy. But then, who could possibly fathom what was going on in his fat head?

One evening – Levin was overdue by now – I came home and spied in the dark, cowering at the front door, a figure which in its miserable shabbiness reminded me of Margot. It was her mother. Dieter wasn't at home. What else could I do but invite the woman in? She lived in a neighbouring village, but had long since broken off all contact with her daughter and had only just learnt of her death from the police. She gave me a stare full of reproach. Apprehensively, I said I was sorry, but I was only the owner of the house.

I had to make tea for her and lend her a supply of handkerchiefs. Frau Müller told me that the father of her illegitimate daughter was dead. When she was only fifteen, Margot was already in with the hash-smoking crowd, and she ended up going on to hard drugs. She went into a home for withdrawal treatment, ran away from there, was picked up as a child prostitute, mended her ways under the wing of a social worker and started training as an apprentice seamstress. When she repeatedly absented herself without any excuse from the workshop, she was kicked out. After this relapse, the whole business started up again. In the end, Frau Müller wanted nothing more to do with her daughter.

Hadn't I heard this kind of tale frequently before?

Fortunately, Dieter arrived shortly after. Now it was his turn to listen to bitter accusations. When, several hours later, he joined me in the conservatory, he was every bit as shattered as I was.

The next day, a telegram arrived. 'AM IN MOROCCO. EVERY-THING FINE. LOVE, LEVIN.' Dieter read it, too, and shook his head. 'Some way to treat a lady.'

I couldn't give a hoot. Without troublemakers, my house was a haven of peace. I had a burning urge to indulge myself. Day after day, I brought back from Heidelberg some object to brighten the place up: sumptuous bunches of flowers and perfumed candles, silk cushions and an exquisite carpet.

Each evening, Dieter and I dined together, taking turn about with the kitchen duties. I caught myself sometimes dolling myself up a bit for the evening meal and feeling disappointed if he wasn't there before me.

Now and again I fancied choosing wallpaper for the attic rooms, but then I would feel uneasy about setting foot there. Dieter was now living alone upstairs and, to be perfectly frank, I could no longer bring myself to think of him moving out.

One day, there was my brother, standing at the door – fortunately without his family. He stayed only for the one evening, but I was delighted to see him. We had a very close and cosy time, sitting chatting about our childhood, our parents and my wedding. That is, until Bob remarked, 'I'm amazed that Dad ate meat at your reception. Maybe he's got over the shock, who can tell?'

'What shock?'

'Don't tell me Mother has never let you in on it . . .'

I gaped at him. Yet again, our mother had entrusted my brother with secrets that weren't for my ears. Old sores were re-opened. 'Well, come on, out with it!' I demanded.

Our beloved grandfather had been a committed Nazi. We all knew that, but it was never talked about.

Only some years after his death, when my father had gone through the last of his papers, did it dawn on him that he was the son of a criminal. My grandfather had taken part in an experimental euthanasia programme; he had – admittedly under orders – mixed poisonous medicines together for mentally ill patients in the municipal hospital, which sooner or later led to their death. In a coded report, cases were recorded which contained the initials of the victims. Again and again, the phrase came up, 'Decease after being served meatballs'. Apparently, he had prescribed concealing the evil-tasting medication in a spicy meat dish. 'After that discovery, Father became a vegetarian,' said Bob, looking at me expectantly.

I felt my heart racing.

'All you inherited from Grandfather was the big leather armchair, wasn't it?' said Bob. 'I don't want his grandfather clock in the house any more. Knowing you, I'm sure you'd take it.'

I nodded. Probably my family had long since forgotten the little glass phials. 'By the way, just what was it Grandmother died of?' I asked abruptly.

'Shingles, I think,' Bob said quickly, reading my darkest thoughts.

The next visitors were Dorit and the children. It was a mild day, and the two little ones ran around in the garden trying to catch blackbirds. We were able to keep an eye on them from the conservatory.

'Have you got over the shock?' my friend asked.

'To some extent,' I replied, 'but Levin has disappeared.'

'Come again? So soon after the wedding and he's done a runner?' Dorit couldn't believe her ears.

'No, no, I don't think it's that. He went to visit friends in Andalusia, and from there he's gone on to Morocco and hasn't surfaced again so far. Do you think I should be worried?'

'I'd be out of my mind if that was Gero,' Dorit reckoned. 'Levin is still accustomed to the free student life, but, whatever way you look at it, it's pretty outrageous!'

'Dorit, do you think Levin would be a responsible father?'

'You never can tell. But, since you ask, I'll be honest with you – you were determined to have him!'

'Dorit, I don't have any children yet. I could still undo the whole thing.'

'You're a right one – marrying under false pretences! You rake in a fortune and a dream villa and then kick your man out into the street! What am I supposed to think of that?'

She was right, too. If I were to get a divorce, then on moral grounds, I'd have to give up my possessions, otherwise I wouldn't even be holding to my own principles. And yet? 'I'm so taken with this house,' I said.

'I can well understand that,' Dorit retorted. 'I certainly wouldn't hand it over again. Besides, many men change once they have a child, and they grow up at last.'

As it was beginning to get dark, we called Franz and Sarah into the conservatory, where I had set out cocoa and biscuits. 'If only', I thought, 'I could cook for children of my own, wipe runny noses, knit woollen jerseys and now, with Christmas coming up, bake ginger biscuits together with them . . .'

After our little coffee and cocoa round, they took their leave. Dorit had forgotten her yellow silk scarf with the blue nautical design. Fleetingly, I buried my nose in it, sniffing the expensive perfume.

I went to the window, but could see only the rear lights of her car, then I looked at the clock. Where had Dieter got to?

All at once I was conscious of how much time in my life I had spent waiting for men. As an activity, it was hard on the nerves, because I was incapable of putting in the waiting time by doing something sensible, something coherent. How often had I kept a meal warm, taken it out of the oven again to prevent it being ruined, then heated it up again till it was finally cooked away to nothing. Exactly like my mother.

So I didn't start cooking, but without something to do, the waiting just got worse. In my desperation, I cleaned the cat's hairs off my blue sweater with Scotch tape. Repeatedly, I peered out of the window to see whether a headlight beam might be signalling Dieter's approach. He arrived just as I was on the verge of tears, and apologized at once.

'What do you mean, you're late?' I asked. 'I hadn't noticed.'

But I was no good at pretending. Dieter was experienced enough to spot that something was wrong. He took me in his arms and kissed me. We cooked some raclette and afterwards made ourselves comfortable on the sofa. The double beds, both upstairs and downstairs, remained unused.

If it hadn't been for Margot haunting my dreams every night, the days that followed would have been happier than ever before. As far as I was concerned, Levin could go hang. Unfortunately, though, sooner or later, his money was bound to run out . . .

Naturally, this wonderful state of hovering betwixt and

between and putting everything out of my mind couldn't last. After only a week of it, clouds were gathering on the horizon. I came home from work like a shot to the arms of my beloved, but the sight of Dieter waiting for me on the doorstep told me that something was wrong.

Levin had phoned from Morocco. He was being held in prison awaiting trial because he had knocked down an old woman. According to his version of events, she had deliberately thrown herself in front of the Porsche. He should be able to get released on bail and to find a lawyer to represent him in the event of a trial.

'For heaven's sake!' I exclaimed. 'So what happened to the poor woman?'

'Fortunately, not much, a broken arm that should heal all right,' said Dieter. 'Levin asked me to get the money to him as soon as possible. To some extent, it's money for a bribe, so it has to be delivered by hand.'

I nodded; so how much?

They were demanding a horrendous amount. Although I agreed right away and was intending to go to the bank first thing in the morning, I had an uneasy feeling. Why couldn't the money simply be sent by bank transfer to the German embassy?

From Dieter's sad expression, I could see that he would have much preferred to stay with me. Nor could the tiring journey be a pleasant prospect for him. So I withdrew the necessary sum without protest, had it converted into dollars and said my farewells to Dieter. Margot's funeral went ahead without him.

Dorit and Gero Meissen invited me to dinner, since I was now left on my own. The children were already asleep, Gero was enjoying a cigar and radiating a delightful fragrance with it. The window was already hung with Christmassy decorations, and for dessert we had baked apples. Gero was listening to our chatter, but with one ear on the news. When it came to a report about someone wanted by the police, this reminded him of something. 'You'll probably take me for a right old gossip-monger, Hella,' he said, 'but I think you probably ought to hear something I picked up recently on the Viernheim grapevine.'

I was always eager to hear what scandal Gero heard from his regular pub evenings with his cronies.

'The Graber family always was a topic for conversation in Viernheim, so naturally the gossip hasn't stopped short of the grandson. Not that I've ever heard anything nasty about your Levin – but the company he kept wasn't always the most select.'

I pricked up my ears. This was going to be about Dieter.

'I know he has a criminal record,' I said.

'But have you any idea why?'

'Drugs?'

'Well, that too,' said Gero, relishing this and letting me dangle on the hook. 'But the main thing your lodger was done for was grievous bodily harm.'

So there was some truth in what Levin had been going on about after all. As far as I was concerned, Dieter had always appeared to be a gentle, peaceable sort.

'I'm sure that was all a long time ago,' I defended my lover. 'People change, but their oh-so-respectable fellow citizens never forgive and forget.'

Gero protested. 'Hella, I'm only passing on what I've heard. It may well be that he's turned into a pillar of society. All the same, I think you should be rather careful.'

Dorit was watching me eagle-eyed. Thanks to feminine intuition, she had noticed at once that I had got jumpy and red in the face at the very mention of Dieter's name. Gero's words had hit home.

'It's nice to have you just to ourselves again, the way it was in the old days,' Gero went on. Yet, as I was leaving, he said, in a placatory tone, 'Marriage must be suiting you, you're looking good.'

'Yes,' I thought, 'for a few days I've been happy having a man about my house.' It was too late to send Dieter on his way – I had fallen head over heels in love with him, much more deeply than with Levin, in fact.

What grounds could I present for divorce from Levin? First and foremost, his relationship with Margot. But could

I afford to bring this humiliation and my hatred out into the open? The police would then probably take a closer interest in Margot's death. I had no idea whether the case had already been closed. To be on the safe side, Levin should never know that I had watched him and Margot. Apart from that, I fervently hoped that Dieter would never let slip to him that he and I had become lovers. Otherwise, it would be reasonable to assume that this had been going on for some considerable time, so I would have had another motive for letting Margot plunge to her death. Oh, come on, Dieter surely wouldn't be so stupid as to give us away.

And yet – the seeds of mistrust were sown. Dieter had been on the road for four days now; he had phoned briefly once, but I could hardly make out what he said.

One evening, I went up to the upstairs flat, in which, because of Margot, I only set foot when I had to. This was where they had lived together. It was furnished partly with the remainder of Hermann Graber's gruesome old pieces, partly with things trawled up from what other people had thrown out.

Everything directly connected with Margot made my gorge rise. In the bathroom, there were still her sticky hair-spray, her make-up things, her nail varnish. Dieter had left the lot, as if she would be back from a trip at any minute. And what about his things? Tentatively, I opened the bedroom cupboard. Dieter's mustard-coloured tweed trousers with the baggy seat and Margot's little black creation hung cheek by jowl.

In the dusty living room stood two old armchairs, a standard lamp with a frilled shade, a display cabinet with the doors removed, in which the radio and the television set had been housed, and Hermann Graber's enormous writing desk. Cautiously, I pulled out the drawers. One was locked. There was nothing special to be found: cigarettes, catalogues and receipts, photos, scissors and paperclips, envelopes and writing paper – remnants of Levin's grandfather – and a box of chocolates, the brand Levin sometimes brought me.

It was the locked drawer that attracted my interest. Again, as at my wedding, Bluebeard's last wife came to my mind, the one who just had to inspect the forbidden room, even though she, like myself, had a premonition of disaster. In that drawer, I would find the decisive clue to Dieter's character. But at that moment, I simply didn't have the key that fitted.

So, was I going to have to force the drawer with a knife? Had Dieter taken the key with him? What was more likely was that he had hidden it away somewhere. I sat down in one of the sagging armchairs and tried to figure out where someone would conceal a small object like that. Perhaps behind that ugly, tasteless oil painting?

I experienced an incredible surge of triumph as I took down an almost black heath-landscape and discovered the key. Without hunting and grubbing around, I had, like some master sleuth, worked out the great secret by sheer imagination.

Fearfully, I opened the drawer. If anything, I'd rather not have pulled it out at all, I was no longer keen to unmask the secret agent.

My eye fell immediately on the money in the open cigar box. It was all in dollars. And it was exactly half of the amount I had changed.

12

There are days in hospital when you lie there in bed, lonely, with never a visit and no mail; on others, they come in their droves and by evening you are utterly exhausted.

On just such a day, the first to arrive was my former colleague Ortrud who, I have always assumed, can't stand me, because I have always been better at the job than her. Unfortunately, I don't to this day know how much she earns. The boss made such a secret of it that I can only suppose she was given preference over me. What it came down to was that here were two sportswomen who had found each other: the boss was an enthusiastic horsewoman, my colleague a hockey player. Mondays they spent showing each other their bruises. Ortrud's rough handshake came as an unpleasant reminder of her sportiness. 'Hella, what's all this you've been up to?' she said, ridding herself of a bunch of dust-covered everlasting flowers.

I was glad when she left. All the same, I was grateful to her for the tip about the jars of baby-food. In a chemist's shop, there isn't very much in the way of comestibles for everyday use. But it seemed that one could, using Junior Stewed Peaches, decorated with cream and a few fresh berries, prepare a delicious dessert, all this at wholesale trade prices, of course.

'I used to have a friend,' Rosemarie Hirte informed me, 'and she freshened up her dried flowers with hair-spray – CFC-free, naturally.'

Frau Römer, Pavel, Kolya, Dorit and Gero all crammed into our room that day. For the first time, my room-mate received a male visitor, a pharmacist by the name of Schröder.

In the end, the whole crowd was mercilessly hustled off the premises by Dr Kaiser. Afterwards, I was almost too exhausted to go on with my story.

*   *   *

The discovery of the money in Dieter's drawer threw me completely. I concocted a variety of explanations for myself. The most improbable was that what we had here was Dieter's own personal belongings. But it looked more as if he was trying to pull a fast one on me. Only Dieter had spoken to Levin, and the wild story he had spun me just couldn't be true. But if my lover was planning to make off with the cash, he would have taken the whole lot with him. And if he had been telling me a pack of lies, it would all come to light when Levin got back.

The solution to the puzzle was, without doubt, that the pair of them were in cahoots. The story about the woman being knocked down might even be true – it fitted in with Levin's driving habits – and it could also be the case that Dieter had to take the bail money to Morocco. But, where the dollars in the drawer were concerned, there was something fishy going on.

Oh, ingratitude! I cursed. Why did I always get taken for a ride by the same shit-awful characters? It was just as well I hadn't allowed Levin access to my bank account, so there was no legal way he could get his hands on my fortune.

'You'll not get the better of me,' I thought. 'I'm your match any day.' But the very thought that they might be after my blood was horrible. If it came to open warfare, I would surely come off second best; it would be better to act nicely and a little naively. Or should I make the grand gesture and hand over my house and my wealth to Levin?

'Money can change a person's character,' I pondered. 'Material things used to be of less importance to me, I was always much more modest in my requirements.' Yet no sooner had I managed to make something of myself than I realized that I had in fact been mistaken in the past.

The next day, Dieter phoned. It had all gone off smoothly, they were already in the North African exclave of Ceuta and would be taking the ferry to Algeciras in Southern Spain the next morning.

Levin took over the receiver and rambled on, all cloying devotion. 'Listen, darling, I can understand you being mad at me. But when you hear what I've been through . . . Would you think it awful bad if Dieter and I stayed on here in the South for another few days, just to rest up a bit?'

I pretended to be rather put out and very anxious, and then, quite distinctly, I could hear Levin lighting a cigarette in relief.

So now I had a few days in which to work out my strategy. A second time, I went upstairs. Maybe there were some clues I had overlooked. Tamerlane had scampered up with me and immediately settled in one of the green upholstered arm-chairs, on which he had already scratched a mossy relief.

For a long time, I stood there in the bedroom, gazing at the flannel bedclothes with the tasteless wild rose pattern, probably something Levin's grandmother had bought as the very latest thing in the sixties. When had these last been washed? Although it made me feel ready to throw up, I raised the three-piece mattresses and the wedge-shaped pillow. But this favourite hiding place probably only worked with elderly people, and professionals would have their own safe-deposit at the bank.

Sadly, I couldn't simply repossess my dollars.

Again, I looked through all the papers. The absence of any certificates, documents and health insurance records was an indication that Dieter had a second depository. Besides, all the rest of his worldly goods were so meagre you could have packed them into two suitcases. Nevertheless, I did find a photo of him with his parents and brothers and sisters, a large family, posing stiffly and in their Sunday best. It didn't look as if his parents had possessed a camera of their own to snap their children in all possible everyday life situations, the way it had happened to me at home. Poor people, it was clear.

A hard youth, all right! What right had I to pass judgement on Dieter? All at once, I felt my dollars were of no importance. I loved that man, no matter what he was planning, and he loved me too. I decided to trust my instincts.

Over and over, I pondered whether I should go and see the lawyer. If he was going to come out of it empty-handed,

Levin would hardly be likely to agree to a divorce, but could he stop me?

He most certainly could, especially since I was, for him, an unwelcome accessory. I would have to adopt similar tactics to Hermann Graber's: draw up a will, stating that, in the event of my death, everything was to go to the Red Cross. I determined to go the very next day to the local court and, for the required fee, deposit just such a document. Levin would receive a photocopy of it.

When I arrived home after carrying out this disagreeable duty, I saw the Porsche and the Mercedes standing side by side in the driveway. So, the gentlemen were back. My knees were shaking, so I sat on in the car for a few minutes. Should I throw my arms round Levin, or Dieter, or neither of them?

No matter what, I had to go inside sooner or later. Before I could get my key out, the front door opened and Levin took me in his arms so tightly I was taken aback.

The table was festively decorated (aside from the plastic place mats), candles were burning and there was a smell of hot butter. He had a lot to make up to me, Levin said, pouring me a glass of sherry.

After a hard day at work and a lengthy drive through the November fog, coming into a warm room is naturally always something special. Many was the time I had received other people in this way, but seldom had it happened to me. The delicious sherry on an empty stomach was doing me good, and I looked at Levin with rather more interest. The shiny bronze of his skin was almost as appetizing as the aroma of food.

'Dieter's still steeping in the bath,' said Levin. 'Actually, he didn't want to eat with us, but I didn't think you'd have any objections.'

Bemused, I shook my head and let him fill up my glass again. At my place lay prettily wrapped presents. 'In a minute or two I'm going to be sitting with my lover and my husband at the same table,' I thought. 'Levin doesn't seem to suspect a thing . . .'

Before I could picture the scene properly, Dieter came in,

looking almost as seductively tanned as Levin. Both of them were in the best of spirits. Dieter gave me a kiss on the cheek and then went to have a look at the Beef Wellington in the oven. 'Ready in a minute,' he announced. 'I hope you're hungry!'

Just what were they up to?

We ate and drank, laughed and joked, and it turned out to be a fantastic evening. Of course it was a delight to sit there between two cheerful men full of compliments and hair-raising tales. I unwrapped my presents. Oriental confectionery, attar of roses, Spanish bootees a size too small and an antique silver candlestick. Levin loved spending money.

From Dieter I got a Moroccan kilim-patterned cushion that fitted marvellously into my grandfather's leather armchair. It was just like Christmas. I almost felt a pang of conscience.

So many lovely presents, all bought with my money! I got a little tipsy and became sentimental. It was high time to get off to bed before the whole beautiful evening ended in tears.

My head was spinning. Had they slipped something into my champagne? Hardly, because very soon Levin came into the bedroom and, with a passion he had never previously demonstrated, clasped me to his tanned chest. I have to admit that my resolution only to sleep with Dieter was forgotten in that moment.

The next morning, I had a hangover, but unfortunately that was no excuse for staying off work. The two men were still asleep. With a thick, pounding head, I sat in the kitchen sipping strong coffee. Once again, my situation was in total confusion. As I breakfasted and tried to cure my hangover, Margot sat like a ghost at my side, telling me how, once upon a time she had been shared by the two friends, and that now it was my turn.

Plagued by doubts, I got into my car. Now, in the depths of winter, it was still dark at seven, and everywhere Christmas trees stood in the gardens, illuminated by electric bulbs. As a child, they had always turned my thoughts to the approach of the Christmas holidays and lightened my spirits on my dark way to school. But in more recent years, I had driven reluctantly to the family home in the festive season, preferring to leave this job to my brother, who at least had managed to present our parents with a grandchild. This year, I would celebrate along with two men with criminal records, not in the bosom of my own family. I hadn't made a single step of progress.

The next evening, too, Levin was all affection and consideration. We were on our own. Cautiously, I asked whether the money had been enough.

Levin eyed me attentively. 'Luckily we didn't need it all to buy my release, otherwise we'd have had nothing left for the return trip and the few days' holiday.'

All by-the-way, I asked a few questions about the remand prison, for it seemed more and more improbable to me that anyone would be locked up because of a road accident.

Levin talked about how he had nearly been lynched by the injured woman's relatives and how the police had only just managed to rescue him from the enraged mob.

'How old was the woman?' I asked.

'About thirty, maybe.'

Dieter had talked about an old woman, and that was the first thing that didn't add up. The second was that Levin was considerably more deeply tanned than Dieter. I refrained from expressing my doubts. Maybe my fears were absolutely unfounded after all. Both of them were behaving quite charmingly. Now that Margot was no longer with us – and we never talked about her any more – even Levin's sexual appetite had improved. It was obvious she had had a complete hold over him. Dieter avoided meeting me on my own. It never came to talking things over, far less a renewal of loving exchanges.

As a chemist, I occasionally did my own pregnancy testing, just for fun, and not only since I had been married to Levin. Shortly before Christmas, it was time to give it another try. For the first time in my life, the test came out positive.

Naturally, I was well aware that, in the early stages, the

chances of error were high, and only an ultrasound scan would provide any certainty. But in the meantime, my instincts told me that I really was pregnant. In the mornings, I felt so sick I couldn't eat a thing, but around noon I would be overcome by such a craving for fresh pastry with yellow custard topped off by three cherries that I would rush out without putting on a coat, but just in my white overall, and nip round to the next-door bakery to buy myself four of these tarts.

If I had been confused before, I was now going crazy. Who was the father of the child? I was rejoicing over an absolutely immoral pregnancy, the kind of thing you would expect from a flighty piece like Margot, but not of a Frau Hella Moormann-Graber. I would giggle to myself, have a good cry in the car; I would have loved to tell the whole world, yet I determined to keep it dark for the time being.

The question was whether I should keep this long yearned-for child of two dubious fathers. In earlier times, too, I had had the chance of having a child without having a husband – and had avoided it out of a sense of responsibility (not as strict as all that, mind you, otherwise all that testing would have been unnecessary). Now I had one Daddy too many, and that wasn't right either.

How I would have loved to tell Dorit about my pregnancy, but I felt it was still too soon for that. Only Tamerlane offered himself as a psychiatrist, and I called on his services frequently. To be on the safe side, I didn't let a drop of alcohol pass my lips, squeezing oranges instead (and bringing the juice straight back up again), and took long walks in the fresh air.

Finally, as if under some neurotic impulse, I thought, 'The first living creature I come across at home is the one I'm going to tell my secret to.' In the fairy tale, that would have been a cat or a dog, but I had one of the two men in mind. And it was only Tamerlane, rubbing himself against my legs. The Porsche was parked in front of the house, but there was no sign of either Levin or Dieter. I went up the stairs, but the top flat was empty too. In the end, I summoned up all my courage and went into the attic. Levin was standing at the fateful window, and he was crying.

I tiptoed up behind him and put my arm round his waist. The sight of a man in tears has always made me melt like chocolate in a *bain-marie*. 'She didn't feel a thing,' I said. 'She lost consciousness right away.'

Levin showed no reaction. Briefly, he blew his nose. 'Where's my stag?' he demanded.

'Who?' I asked, confused.

It transpired that he meant that massive old wardrobe with the carvings of capercaillies and stags that the young couple had carted off. His grandmother, he wailed, had always told him tales of the animals of the forest, inspired by these carved figures. I comforted him and kept my maternal joys from him.

Frau Hirte chortled, 'So tomorrow I'll get to hear which stag was the dominant male, will I?'

13

Actually, Rosemarie isn't all that bad as a room-mate; when I think of those whining women I come across in the day-room, I even feel as if I've won first prize. I'm sorry for having been rather snooty about her at first.

She seems to get out in the fresh air a lot, either walking other people's dogs or pushing that man about in his wheel-chair. Because of all this, she has educated herself to be something of an amateur ornithologist, extremely well versed in those few birds that still inhabit our forests. Recently she was telling me how, a hundred years ago, some loony tried to introduce to North America all the species of birds that feature in the collected works of Shakespeare. Since that time, there are star-lings there.

But of course I was able to pass on much more interesting titbits to her, like, for example, the story of my pregnancy.

We were coming up to Christmas, I was expecting a child and could at long last indulge in a long suppressed craving for kitsch and sentimentality. I had inherited my grandparents' Christmas tree decorations, because my mother had put into practice her own individual idea of what a fashionable tree should look like, with pink or lilac bows. For the first time, I opened the little chest full of fragile lametta, angel's hair, glass bells, candle holders caked with wax, wooden teddy bears, Little Red Riding Hoods and skaters all in the most delicate fretwork, not forgetting Grandmother's gold papier mâché Christmas fairy. Dieter and Levin looked on as I unpacked all these treasures. Most of them were intended for the tree, but the carved carol singers and the little smoking man from the Erzgebirge area of the south-east could already be set up during Advent.

Levin had a feeling for nostalgia, so he brewed up a punch out of red wine, cloves and sugar. The concoction went straight to your head, and the two men went all silly.

I hadn't had a good look at the dear little golden Christmas fairy for ages. As a child, I believed this figure to be the Christ-child in person. The delicate face and tiny hands were fashioned out of wax. A pleated dress of stiff, slightly worse for wear, gold papier mâché made the angel sparkle magnificently and helped her to stand firmly upright.

'What did she call it?' Dieter asked. 'Papier hashy?' Levin burst out in uncontrollable fits of laughter. Dieter giggled along with him and soon neither could stop.

'Our papier hashy angel's getting peeved,' said Levin. 'Just look at how the veins under her golden hairline are starting to bulge. There's an analytical mind at work there.'

They kept calling the fairy that for the whole evening. Under normal circumstances, I'd have had a good go at the red wine punch as well, but my special condition held me back. Which explained why I wasn't in the mood for fun.

Their joke had a special meaning, which I guessed right away: they had used my dollars to put through a major deal, and Levin hadn't been stuck in any dreary cell at all, but had been having fun surfing somewhere. Racked by doubts, I looked from one to the other. 'Which one is the father of my child?' The question wouldn't stop running through my mind. According to all my calculations, each of them had a roughly equal chance of becoming a father in the coming year.

'Your papier hashy angel's going to bed,' I said. 'You can drink to your big successes without me. But don't imagine for a moment you can take me for a complete fool.'

I asked the fairy, 'What am I supposed to do? Why do I always do everything wrong in life?' The fairy stood to attention and quoted from Schiller's *Wallenstein*, 'If you put not your life at stake, never shall life be yours to win.' Although I was asleep, I could feel the heavenly messenger sprinkling white powder over me like snowflakes. 'Snow-flake, coke-flake, snow is falling, snow on snow.'

When, the next morning, I glanced into the still messy kitchen, the sight once again brought me close to vomiting. Had Levin mixed some powder into my food this time? Whatever it was, I looked out the photocopy of my will and left it lying demonstratively on the filthy kitchen table.

At work, I had no time to sit and think as a rule. Quite apart from those busy people who want to pick up their prescriptions in a hurry, there were a few chatty regulars. As a rule, these were old, lonely folk, whose one break in the daily routine was an outing to the doctor's and the chemist's. I was well aware that my job had a social function: not only advice, but also a sympathetic ear was what they were looking for. Whereas I never dodged them, my boss was only too happy to disappear from sight the moment those persistent moaners hove into view. At that, even my sporty colleague, Ortrud, would murmur gloatingly, 'Hella, it's your turn.'

Occasionally, I would have to listen patiently to quite absurd tales, often to do with 'nasty' relatives. Her daughter-in-law, one old woman told me, was trying to kill her off, more than once counting out her drops wrongly. Actually I had no doubt that in certain families there would be attempts to *corriger la fortune*, and that, within the intimacy of a shared household, the odds must indeed be favourable.

Mostly, it's mothers who turn up in the shop, to collect medicines for sick children, grannies and husbands, or the pill for themselves. One exception was Pavel Siebert, a joyless, middle-aged man who lived nearby and took care of all the shopping for his family. In an effort to cheer him up, my boss had brought him along that time I had thrown our party.

He was a taciturn man, pleasant enough, but not one for engaging you in conversation. As time went on, and judging by the prescriptions he brought in, we had deduced that his wife was undergoing psychiatric treatment. From Dorit, my inquisitive boss had heard that the poor woman was suffering from psychosis and was plagued by bouts of paranoid hallucinations.

I was on my own in the shop when this unfortunate, but none the less good-looking man came in shortly before closing time. On this occasion, he seemed in a rather more approachable frame of mind.

'How is your wife?' I inquired boldly.

He gave me a wary look. 'She's in hospital for the time being.'

'There are people who are worse off than I am,' the thought flashed through my mind. How on earth did he manage to do a job and look after his ailing children at the same time, I asked as I glanced at the prescription, which showed he had a 'Dr' before his name.

He was an editor in an academic publishing house and could do part of his work at home, he told me. 'I can manage the housework pretty well,' he said, not without a trace of pride. 'Only very seldom are there problems in that respect.' And, by the way, he was sorry, but he had forgotten my name, even though he had visited my house once.

I found that understandable. 'Moormann, Hella Moormann,' I said. 'Or to be more precise, Hella Moormann-Graber.'

Ah, yes, he said, that reminded him of the announcement of my marriage in the paper. 'My wife made a joke at the time, about grabbing the woman from the moors,' he laughed brightly.

I was almost sorry he knew about my marriage at all. But I was annoyed at his wife. There she was, holed up in the loony bin, leaving her husband to look after the household and making stupid jokes about people from the moors.

I set about closing up shop. 'I'm sure my husband is already waiting impatiently to make another grab at his bog-trotter,' I said grumpily.

Pavel Siebert realized at once that I didn't think much of his witticism. He gave me an apologetic look, and suddenly it was clear that we liked each other.

On my way home, I was so thoroughly overcome by fear that

127

I felt the desire to turn round and drive back to the sanctuary of my chemist's shop. How had Levin reacted to the will?

My husband was waiting for me, looking very grave and profoundly hurt. The will was lying on the table in front of him. 'Is this supposed to be some kind of a joke? If it is, it's a poor one.'

'It's something I learned from your grandfather,' I said. 'There's no point in doing me in, for you'd come out of it empty-handed.'

Levin stared at me open-mouthed. Only now had the penny dropped, and he was deeply offended. 'Have you gone completely mad? I do everything I can to treat you with love and affection, and you seriously believe I would try to bump you off? That's hardly a basis for us to go on living together.'

Now I was sorry for him, and I regretted what I had done. It was indeed true that, since his trip, he had been nicer to me. But I wasn't going to give in.

'So why am I your "paper hashy angel"?' I demanded.

How on earth could I have taken that seriously, a simple little play on words, two chaps who had had a drink or three . . . ?

'I took it very seriously indeed. You both used my money to fund some bit of dirty business,' I said. 'You're trying to get rich on the suffering and death of young people.'

Now it was Levin's turn to cut up nasty. 'What do you mean, your money?' he shouted. 'It never was your money, every penny of it comes from my family. But supposing I really was some kind of a monster, then I could torture you now and force you to make out a new will while I watched. And that would be you signing your own death warrant.'

'I'm neither old nor sick, nor do I have false teeth yet. You'd have to come up with something pretty special so as not to be condemned as a murderer.'

It was obvious what was going on in Levin's mind. 'You could always fall out of an attic window; suicide as a result of severe depression.'

'Nobody would buy that,' I said. 'I've never suffered from depressions in my life. All my friends would testify to that.'

'I could make you write a farewell note,' said Levin. 'One that would be bound to convince your friends.'

We stared at each other, our eyes filled with hate. I was at the end of my tether. Since I could think of nothing else to come back with on the subject, I burst into tears. 'I'm pregnant,' I sobbed.

'You're what? You're having your period, that's what. I know only too well how hysterical that can make you.'

I rushed into the bedroom to carry on crying on my bed. Shortly afterwards, I heard the front door slamming and the Porsche roaring off.

Levin didn't come home all night.

The next morning, still no sign of either the car or its driver. In my dressing-gown, I went into the kitchen to put the kettle on. Without an audience, I had lost the urge to cry. At the very moment I was throwing up my camomile tea into the sink, Dieter came in. I wiped my mouth on some kitchen roll and sat down at the table, breathing heavily. Dieter gave me a searching look. We were both ill at ease.

'I've already heard you several times, being sick in the mornings,' said Dieter, a note of anxiety, and at the same time a trace of suggestiveness, in his voice. He squeezed a lemon and made me sniff the fresh tang. Then he went to the fridge, took out a can of cola and poured me out a glass. 'Secret recipe,' he recommended. I drank it and, amazingly, the icy, disgusting concoction did me good. In a rare affectionate gesture, Dieter stroked my hair and left.

For all that he normally slept next to me, my husband had never so much as noticed my early-morning retchings. Dieter, on the other hand, had detected it from the floor above. But if Dieter had recognized the signs of pregnancy, then he would also have to take into consideration the possibility that he himself could be the father. Or did men never check back on these things?

That day, I had an appointment with the gynaecologist. In a fever, I waited for his verdict.

After that, I couldn't get to Dorit's fast enough.

'And what has the happy father-to-be to say about it?' she asked.

'He doesn't know anything yet about how happy he should be. You're the first. After all, I did promise.'

'I am indeed honoured,' said Dorit. 'But when you tell him, do pretend he's the first to know.'

Now we had a great deal to talk about, things like the way I'd feel and the weird cravings pregnancy arouses, a topic that had always been close to Dorit's heart, but one she had, out of a sense of tact, seldom foisted on me.

However, since I was neither dancing for joy nor demanding champagne so that I could then smash the glasses against the wall, she inquired, with a foreboding bordering on suspicion, whether all was not well with Levin.

'Oh, no,' I said, 'but I feel so constantly awful, and I can't really believe it myself yet.'

'That'll get better with each day that passes,' said Dorit. 'The sickness will go after the third month, it'll just vanish, and as your tummy gets bigger and rounder, the dream will turn into reality.'

I stayed a long time with my friend, with the result that Gero was the second to hear the news. He gave me a kiss, and, with a wink to his wife, said, 'I hope Dorit's not going to use this as an excuse to talk me into a third one!'

She laughed. 'Now that you mention it . . .'

Finally, I drove off homewards. Would Levin be there? I wondered. And if he was, how would he take it?

There sat the two men in the kitchen, as if nothing had happened, and a meal was ready, nice as you like. 'I bought a deep-frozen Polish goose today, for Christmas,' said Dieter.

'And I was at the doctor's,' I said, bold as brass. 'I'm two months gone.'

Levin gave me a disbelieving look.

Dieter immediately fetched the champagne, which I could have done without. Altogether against my new-found principles, I took a sip and enjoyed at last being once again the centre of attention. As if our bitter altercation had never happened, we all three got on marvellously that evening.

The gold papier mâché angel stood on a palm tree in the conservatory and gave us her blessing.

Unfortunately, I was the one who shattered the peace. I had this uncanny feeling that Margot was lying in the hammock, watching us; in reality it was the cat who was luxuriating there. Margot, who had also had a child – exactly whose was a question equally difficult to unravel as the present one – was haunting me.

'I wish you'd stop this boozing!' I yelled suddenly, and the two men gawped at me, startled.

Tamerlane, too, leapt out of the hammock, which continued to swing violently for some time.

As so often before, I withdrew, but not before giving orders that the kitchen had to be cleared up.

Quite out of the blue, and through none of his doing, a second trip became a bitter necessity for Levin. He received a telephone call from Vienna to say that his mother had had a bad car accident. It was perfectly clear from Levin's grief-stricken expression that this story was no fabrication. He didn't ask me for any cash, but naturally I provided him with a ticket for his flight and changed some money into Austrian Schillings. I was all for buying him a coat, but, as a matter of principle, Levin never wore anything but short jackets.

Should I go with him? I wondered. At that moment, flying was the last thing I wanted. All I knew of Levin's mother was that she was an ardent admirer of the works of Annette von Droste-Hülshoff, after whom she had intended naming the daughter she had so long yearned for. When, to her disappointment, it turned out to be a boy, it had fallen to the writer Annette's childhood friend Levin Schücking to provide a name for him.

It was five days before Christmas Eve, and I had taken two weeks' holidays from work. It was with some apprehension that I realized I was now alone in the house with Dieter. No doubt he would be keen to have the whole matter aired.

We were still at our evening meal, which we were having by the light of the Advent candles, when Dieter heaved a

131

deep sigh, as if by way of an introduction, so that I couldn't help asking, 'What's up?'

'It's no easy matter for me,' said Dieter, his gentle voice now heavy with sadness, 'to sit looking on at how happy you are with Levin. Those days you spent with me have been forgotten, it seems.'

I assured him that the contrary was true.

Personal feelings were of secondary importance, Dieter insisted, and all that mattered now was the welfare of the child. As he spoke, he looked at me with an expression full of such misery that, quite spontaneously, I threw my arms round him.

'We're going to be on our own for a few days,' I began. 'And I'm on holiday . . .' I felt thoroughly irresponsible.

'But you're pregnant, remember,' Dieter admonished me.

The devil was in me. 'The child is yours,' I said.

Dieter knew exactly what was expected of him. He embraced me and kissed me and gave all the signs of genuine delight. 'When are you going to tell Levin?' he asked.

'That's really not on at the present,' I fended him off. 'I mean, his mother might well be on her deathbed.'

That evening, I went to bed with Dieter and the jealous Tamerlane. I was surprised at myself, but it was simply wonderful.

14

There were some things Rosemarie couldn't quite get straight. Like the business with the children who, from time to time, ran wild in our peaceful room. Which ones belonged to whom?

Dorit, I explained, had two children, Franz and Sarah, who were roughly the same ages as Pavel's two, Kolya and Lene.

'What kind of names are these?' grumped Rosemarie. 'But that's not really what I'm driving at. So Kolya and Lene are the children of Pavel and the crazy Alma – am I right?'

I nodded.

'And the littlest one, that pain in the neck?'

'He's called Niklas.'

She growled. 'What a shambles! Would you like a squirt of perfume? Now, come on, get on with the story, will you!'

When Levin phoned from Vienna, he was sobbing loudly. His mother was now in a coma, and things looked far from good. They were allowing him into the intensive care ward for only a few minutes at a time. I tried to give him some comfort and courage, but it was perfectly understandable that, in such a situation, my words were not even getting through to him.

Whenever, in the early stages of our relationship, I tried to cajole something out of Levin, I usually succeeded, because basically he was no more than a child, glad to let slip his little secrets. Only about 'men's affairs' did he betray nothing. Dieter was different, consistent in his silence. I learned next to nothing at all about his family.

'How many brothers and sisters have you?' I asked.

'Too many.'

'Are your parents still alive?'

'If they haven't died . . .'

Still, as we lay cuddling up close and lovingly on the sofa, I persisted in my attempts to find out something about Dieter's past. 'I heard, quite by chance, that you've done time for assault,' I said tentatively, snuggling up even closer.

'Uhuh,' said Dieter. Then, finally, he admitted, 'I hit someone. Twice.'

I gave a vicarious shudder.

On the first occasion, a junkie had grassed on him. This led on to Dieter admitting to having dealt in drugs in the past. Apparently he had inflicted more than just a bloody nose on his victim. Confessing to the second assault proved to be agony for Dieter. As I already knew, Margot had got pregnant and was married to Dieter. He wasn't looking forward to this child, and he locked Margot in, to make sure that she had no opportunity to get her hands on heroin. One night, she had abseiled down from the second floor and had made off. Days later, he discovered her streetwalking in Frankfurt's west end. Dieter picked her up, brought her home and gave her such a hammering she had to be treated in hospital.

'But there was no harm done to the kid,' said Dieter. 'I made sure of that.'

That I couldn't understand. 'How can anybody blow his top and yet still spare the pregnant woman's belly?'

'I don't know either,' said Dieter lamely.

So after that, she stopped shooting, but he went on peddling, as I understood it.

Once you were into the racket, it seemed you couldn't get out of it just like that.

'And what did the two of you buy in Morocco?'

'Just some dope, honest. Not a single gram of heroin. There isn't any to be had there anyway.'

Nevertheless, I learned that Margot had provided him with an alibi for his one big-time deal; the price she demanded for her false statement was not money, but marriage.

I would have liked to ask him next about what had happened to half of my dollars, but I didn't dare.

* * *

There followed a few days of peace and tranquillity. Together, we went to hear Bach's Christmas Oratorio in St Mark's in Weinheim, and after that, late in the evening, we baked some Nuremberg gingerbread. And at last I had a companion for my walks through the Odenwald and the Palatinate. Loveliest of all were the vine-clad paths along the hilltops that led northwards to Heppenheim, or to Schriesheim in the south. Startled pheasants would flutter up from the bramble bushes, there were quinces, which thrive in this area, rotting in the allotments and giving off their irresistible fragrance, and ivy climbing up the fruit trees, and the dim, misty days were like some fairy tale, so enchanting – summer never had anything like this to offer. Once we went for a stroll through the Christmas Market in Heidelberg, then, back home, we roasted the chestnuts we had bought and played chess. Although Dieter had to eat all the chestnuts and the home-baked biscuits on his own – to be on the safe side, I was sticking to plain pastry fingers and chilled cola – that was a brief interval of wonderful peace. I knew all too well that it couldn't last.

Practically every day, Dieter pleaded with me to get a divorce; after all, it was his child, not Levin's. Unlike me, he seemed to entertain not the slightest doubt.

In the paper, I happened to come across an item that said: 'A spouse's legal entitlement to inheritance is nullified in such cases where the testator has filed a court application for divorce prior to decease and this petition has already been served on the partner in marriage.'

No doubt Dieter had studied this same expert judgement and therefore was aware that a husband could not inherit his wife's possessions if, at the time of her death, a petition for divorce had already been filed in a court. I eyed him closely. Was he perhaps intending to make himself my heir?

Suddenly, I could control myself no longer. 'The two of you blew only half of the money,' I said. 'Why have you been lying to me?'

Dieter went pale. 'Did Levin tell you that?' he asked, shaken.

'Yes,' I lied.

135

He had put aside half of my dollars for me, he said.

'So why did you con the money out of me in the first place?'

'It was Levin's idea. He's in debt to me.'

'But Levin has money of his own!'

That had him. 'I swear to you, Hella, I'm not going to let him influence me any more. I was dead against asking you for money, right from the start.' Dutifully, he scuttled off and brought back my bundle of dollars.

'It's not just a question of the money,' I said, nevertheless counting it just to teach him a lesson. 'What I hate, though, is being deceived.'

Dieter nodded. 'As of now, this is the start of a new life,' he said. 'I'm not that crazy about money either. As far as I'm concerned, you can give it all to Levin when you get divorced.'

'I wouldn't dream of it,' I said. 'But quite apart from that, I can't very well greet him with the news – when he gets back, straight from his mother's deathbed – that you're to be my new husband, and the father of my child into the bargain. If I did, he'd end up doing himself in!'

To top it all, while we were talking about him, Levin himself phoned again. He was in the depths of despair. It was enough to melt a heart of stone. 'The worst of it is,' he finally managed to bring out between sobs, 'I can't tell my mother any more that we're happily married and expecting a baby!'

Christmas was two days away. Dieter had bought a small tree; he was looking forward to the celebrations. He had never had it so good, he told me, a comfortable home, a loving woman, the prospect of a child. He said he had made the final break with his old acquaintances from his drug-dealing days. Because of me, he had become a new man.

Dorit had little spare time during these busy days. Where there are two small children around, Christmas preparations take on a higher priority. During our telephone calls she was breathless and harassed, and there was little point in trying to explain the business of the two fathers now. But Levin's wails did give me the idea of phoning my own parents and

136

announcing to them that they could look forward to the joys of grandparenthood in the New Year.

'We've been waiting a long time for this news,' was my mother's retort. 'I mean, you have been married for over six months.'

I kept a hold of myself. 'Well, for once in my life, I've lived up to your expectations,' was all I said.

My father took over the conversation; he had been listening in. 'I hope everything's going along fine,' he said.

Even this pious wish niggled me. 'I'm not as ancient as that yet. I can still have children for another ten years,' I insisted.

'It wasn't aimed at your youthfulness,' said Father gallantly, 'but at your young husband.'

I hung up. They weren't going to hear again from me in a hurry, and I certainly had no intention of making the customary Christmas and New Year's calls.

Two hours later, my brother Bob was on the line. The old folks had already put him in the picture. 'Congratulations,' he said. 'What do you say if we come to see you on New Year's Eve? I'll bring Grandfather's clock along.'

Normally, I would have been delighted at the prospect of Bob's visit – especially if he came without his wife – but for the moment I wanted to be alone with my two men and my condition. My brother would have sniffed out complications which could not yet be foreseen.

'Oh, Bob,' I said, 'that's really kind of you, but I'm feeling rotten the whole time. I want to make the most of the holiday period to have a long lie-in in the mornings and do as little in the kitchen as possible – the very smell of an onion frying makes me want to throw up. I'd be a useless hostess.'

And that was how I squandered the opportunity of having my brother in the house at the very time I could really have done with his presence. Those New Year celebrations will haunt my memory for as long as I live.

When, on Christmas Eve, I returned home after an exhausting shopping trip, there was a note on the table. Levin had asked to be picked up at Frankfurt Airport; his mother had died during the night. Dieter had set off right away. I had knocked my ankle against a shopping trolley, jammed a finger in the tailgate of the car, and now I was standing there by the fridge with my heavy carrier bags. No doubt the two gentlemen would expect a meal to be ready for them.

It was an emaciated, despondent Levin who returned home, expecting to be embraced and rocked in my arms like a child. He drank a little tea and then lay sniffling in the hammock, while Dieter fixed the Christmas tree in its stand and I vacuumed up the pine needles. Finally, I started hanging my grandparents' decorations on it. There was a smell of the forest about the place. Levin brought the record player and one of his favourite records, 'Orpheus and Eurydice', out to the conservatory.

'She is gone, and gone for ever, all my joy, alas, is flown!' we heard at full blast. Up till then, I had always fantasized on hearing these sounds that the lost one was myself, and the heart-rending lament was directed at me. Now it was meant for his mother – wasn't that a bit incestuous?

Dieter appeared not to follow my train of thought, absent-mindedly fixing a star to the top of the tree.

I would have much preferred turning on the radio and tuning in to some schmaltzy American Christmas ballad, but instead, the air was rent by *'Vain expectation! Nowhere, to cheer me, consolation, nowhere relief.'*

Levin was accompanying the words with such whimperings, I could hardly make them out any more. How could I have tortured him further with plans for separation, at this of all times?

A thoroughly melodramatic little coffee session followed.

'If there can be any consolation at all,' said Levin, 'then it's the baby. One loved one dies, but another is born. If it's a girl, then we've just got to name her after my mother.'

I knew she was called Auguste. 'Did she have any other name?' I asked tentatively, for the first time hoping for a son.

'Of course,' said Levin. 'Auguste Friederike. And by the

way, people called her Gustel. That's really quite nice, isn't it?'

'I'd go along with Friederike,' I said, and noticed Dieter twitching.

After dinner, we lit the candles and sat rather at a loss around our tree. Dieter brought some wine and, after five glasses of it, Levin became euphoric. 'Next year, there'll not be just the two of us,' he said, overlooking Dieter at my side. 'Our child will shout with joy when it sees the burning candles and the brightly coloured decorations.'

Dieter swallowed hard and then said, 'And in two years' time, our child will be walking.'

Levin paid no heed to the possessive adjective. He took another drink, embraced me and insisted that this was the happiest Christmas of his life, but five minutes later he was again describing it as the saddest.

Dieter said not another word but just carried on drinking. I was feeling more and more afraid, and didn't like the look of either of them. Outside, it had started to rain, not, of course, to snow, the way one hoped for year in year out. From the radio came the sounds of bells and children's choirs.

'Our child is going to learn to play the piano,' said Levin. 'Hella, do you think it will be musical? After all, my father was an organist.'

I squinted across at Dieter, who abruptly grabbed at the nearest Christmas ball on the tree and hurled it at the large conservatory window.

Levin stiffened, while I dropped my piece of gingerbread.

But Dieter hadn't finished at that. One ball after another crashed against the window pane and exploded into sparkling shards.

I tried to stop Dieter, but Levin held me back. Quietly, he said, 'The best thing is if we disappear. There's no saying what he'll do next!'

It didn't seem right to me to leave Dieter on his own with the Christmas tree and its lighted candles, but Levin pulled me into the bedroom and locked the door. Not only that, but he pushed the chest of drawers against the door to form a pretty solid barricade. I was sweating blood. 'I'm sure he won't do anything to harm us,' I whispered.

Levin seemed not to give a thought as to why Dieter was going on the rampage like that, while I knew all too well the reason for it. We could hear the most blasphemous oaths and finally a tremendous crash and a seemingly endless tinkling of glass. I suspected that one of the big conservatory windows had been smashed. When all had been silent for some time, we crept out. Dieter was no longer there. But the conservatory looked like a battlefield. 'We've got to get the plants into the rooms where it's warm,' I said. 'They'll freeze in temperatures like this.'

The rest of Christmas Eve was spent lugging plant pots and tubs, without Levin being plagued with the slightest doubt as to whether this heavy work was good for me. Lastly, we swept up the splinters and shards of broken glass and Levin tried to patch up the enormous hole with plastic bags and pieces of cardboard. It would keep out the wind and rain for the time being, but any burglar would have no trouble just walking straight in. How on earth were we to find a glazier on the twenty-fifth of December? We shelved that problem and went off to bed. Levin fell asleep at once, while I could only lie there, furious and exhausted, letting out tearless sniffs and snorts.

As morning dawned, it also dawned on me that I was not an altogether innocent party to this disaster. There was nothing else for it, I would have to decide, to choose the one father or the other. After Dieter's fit of maniacal rage, I wondered whether he deserved to be favoured: he had disqualified himself. And how would he react if I turned him down? I didn't dare to imagine.

On that Christmas morning, Tamerlane stared at me reproachfully: nothing was in its rightful place, everywhere he turned, plants in large pots stood in his way. Since there was no one else to listen to me, I treated my cat to a speech. 'If you were a dog,' I told him, 'I would take you off right now for a long walk. And besides, you could stand guard at nights, to make sure no burglars get in. You just can't depend on men.'

The two of them were asleep. I drank some tea and ate a sandwich, quite surprisingly without it making me feel ready to vomit. Then I put on warm clothes and got into the car. I drove out for a bit into the Odenwald and – with not another soul in sight – went on a long winter hike to clear my head. But even with a clear head I was incapable of arriving at any significant decisions. I gave Dieter a sound cursing and scolded Levin for being such a mummy's boy. 'Only you matter,' I said to my child.

When I finally got back home, all rosy cheeked and with warm feet, there was a note from Dieter on the table: 'A glazier will be round at three to measure up.' In addition he – for Levin could be ruled out – had knocked out the dangerous jagged shards remaining in the window frame and cleared up the rest of the splinters of Christmas balls from the tree and glass from the window and dumped them in the dustbin.

Levin emerged from his bed. 'I'm sorry, Sweetheart,' he said. 'I had a fair bit of sleep to catch up on.'

'Sure. That's all right.'

'Can you remember what it was that made Dieter go berserk like that?' he asked.

I shook my head.

Levin asked if there was any coffee. As I put water on to boil, I noticed that Dieter had placed the frozen goose next to the oven, but since it would take at least fourteen hours to thaw out, we could pretty well forget Christmas dinner for today.

'Where is Dieter anyway?' asked Levin.

I had no idea either.

The glazier arrived, gave a disapproving shake of the head and drew his own conclusions. 'And on Christmas Eve, too,' he muttered. 'How can anything like that happen? It must have been nothing short of sheer brute force!'

I looked thoughtfully at this wise man. He was right. You could never smash a window pane with a mere paper-thin Christmas ball. Dieter must have got Hermann Graber's sledgehammer out of the cellar, and so the whole thing could no longer be excused as an unpremeditated act.

141

Despite the miserable weather, I wrapped up warm and took myself off outside, but I couldn't make up my mind to go for another walk. In the garden, I spread a plastic carrier bag on the damp garden seat and sat down. A friendly robin settled right in front of me. I didn't budge, and it watched me carefully with its little black eyes.

As a child, I had been deeply impressed by the folk tale of 'Yorinde and Yoringel', where hundreds of caged nightingales are in fact young maidens under a witch's magic spell. Ever since then, I've always known that birds are animals like any other, but they are also the messengers of our soul. In countless songs, poems and fairy stories, birds feature as symbols of good or evil forces, as harbingers of news, as omens of death and disaster or of hope and new love. In the light of the poetry in these songs, I had a notion that there existed another kind of love which I had been hitherto denied.

Many a time I had even wondered whether I wouldn't rather have been an animal, and if so, which one? If I had the choice, then I would want to be able to fly. In the early days, I thought of being a bat; there are all different sorts, but they all have something devilish, demonic about them. With their big pointed ears, their slightly protruding eyes and their sharp teeth, they are heralds of darkness, bloodsuckers. Yet, when, on a warm summer evening in southern lands, you watch them flitting about with that infinite lightness and agility, then you feel the urge to join them. That's just the way it is with me about my favourite birds, swallows. What they have in common with bats is that they labour so hard to feed themselves and their brood. Did I really want to have to slave away all my life, just to have enough to eat?

So rather than that, my choice fell on a bird of prey. Not an eagle, but a buzzard; not for me, that monumental, stately flight. Who has not, on a day during a holiday, lain in the grass watching a bird of prey circling overhead? High above us and our problems, it drifts through the blue air, detached, rapt. Only now and then it plummets down on a mouse, for his majesty has to eat, too.

Maybe, some day, I would manage to lead the life of a bird of prey, concerned with nothing other than carrying the

142

captured mouse back to the nest and to my young. There would be a second buzzard circling beside me – no other birds can survive at such altitudes. I would be a protected species, I could have all the mice I wanted, and I would never so much as lay a claw on lambs.

15

At long last he had found a young man to do the gardening, Pavel told me during an evening visit. All right, his knowledge of German was pretty thin, but against that, he was intelligent and willing to work. 'He can't help it if he's illiterate; if only I had just a little more time . . .'

What did he look like, I wanted to know. 'A handsome young lad,' replied Pavel.

Delighted at the prospect, I began to wonder whether we might ask at the Adult Education Centre about suitable teaching materials.

'Careful,' said Rosemarie, once we were on our own. 'Not another one, surely!'

That annoyed me. My conversations with Pavel were none of her business. Previously, she had at least turned a deaf ear or gone out into the corridor just out of courtesy.

But there was no stopping her now, and she launched into what amounted to a homily. I formed a wrong picture of most people, she told me, and that was bound to end in tears . . .

'Well, I've no illusions about you,' I thought. 'You're a shrivelled old maid without a past and with no future.' And then I went straight back to spinning my tale of skulduggery.

My parents phoned, full of the festive spirit. 'We haven't heard from you in ages,' they claimed.

Somewhat brusquely, I wished them the compliments of the season. 'If you only knew,' I thought to myself.

My boss called, too, humming and hawing for a bit. She was wondering whether I might stand in for a sick colleague for a few days. 'Otherwise, I'm completely on my own in the shop, Hella. I mean, you know how hectic it can get here after the holiday period.'

She was right, of course. Countless people who have eaten, drunk and smoked too much and it hasn't agreed with them. And others who can't cope with the increased emotional demands made on them during the festival of love and come looking for Valium, just like Dorit. To my boss's amazement, I agreed without a murmur. In the secure world of the chemist's shop, I felt better than within my own four walls.

On Boxing Day, however, I was still at home. Dieter put in an appearance again, hardly said a word and set about preparing the goose with all the proper trimmings, red cabbage and dumplings. The atmosphere was dismal. Levin appeared to have no desire to bring up the subject of his friend's outburst, and I certainly wasn't going to. I had to work from the twenty-seventh until the thirtieth, but unfortunately I would be off again on New Year's Eve.

The shop really was taken by storm, as if we were having a closing-down sale. The last to turn up was Pavel Siebert. 'So what have your children caught this time?' I asked as I looked out some fever-reducing suppositories.

'They've both got measles. And over the Christmas holidays of all times!'

I felt really sorry for him. His second problem, he went on in a more confidential tone, was his little daughter's birthday cake. 'I have a recipe there all right,' he said dejectedly, 'but I don't think I dare try my hand at baking.'

This was my big moment! I got quite carried away. On the evening before the red-speckled daughter's birthday, there I was, standing in a strange kitchen, baking a chocolate cake and showing off my skills with marzipan Mickey Mouse figures.

The morose Pavel turned out to be a charming assistant, who insisted on our drinking a toast once the job was done, he in red wine, I in apple juice. More than once, the children, in pyjamas and slippers, tried to storm the kitchen, but their father kept them at bay. 'It's supposed to be a surprise,' he shouted, helping himself to a Minnie Mouse with chocolate ears. Would I, he asked, like to come round the next morning and taste my delicious cake? 'You see, children with measles can't very well invite their friends in. But I'm sure you're immune . . .'

'We'll see,' I said.

Back home, all was silent as the grave. Only Tamerlane jumped up to welcome me. Still, the glazier had already put in a new pane, and one of my men had restored the plants to their proper places, done a thorough cleaning and placed a bunch of yellow roses on the table. Since the heating in the conservatory was still set low and Levin always turned it up full blast, I assumed it was all Dieter's work.

'What am I doing here anyway?' I asked myself despondently. Then I phoned Dorit. 'Today I baked a chocolate cake for a child's birthday,' I told her.

Right away, Dorit's curiosity was roused. 'Aha, old Siebert?' she said. 'Lene goes to the same nursery school as our Sarah. A sweet little thing, and, despite her mad mother, not in the least disturbed.'

'Why is the fellow called Pavel anyway?' I asked.

Apparently his family came from Prague originally. He always came to collect his daughter from nursery. 'I like the man,' said Dorit. 'I've a soft spot for academics, and especially if they have a big bushy beard like Karl Marx.'

I had to laugh. In fact, I really liked the beard, myself. 'Too bad we're both spoken for, and Pavel too. And soon I'm going to be all sticking out in front, and no bushy-bearded stranger will want to bake chocolate cakes with me.'

'Tell you what,' Dorit suggested, 'we could bring in the New Year together. I'm sure my parents would be only too happy to look after the children.'

I had already put off my brother Bob, and I wasn't all that keen on Dorit's idea either. The combination of the whining Levin, the jealous Dieter and alcohol was not the happiest one. But maybe a nice girlfriend and an upstanding citizen like Gero could prove to be my salvation.

* * *

I had just heated up a thin soup for myself and was sitting spooning it up listlessly when Dieter came in. 'I'm sorry about all that,' he said grumpily, 'but things can't go on like this. You've got to tell Levin I'm the father.'

I didn't answer.

'There's no point in going easy on him any longer,' said Dieter. 'He's in mourning just now anyway, so we might as well get it all over with in one fell swoop.'

Completely drained, I looked at him, while he stared grimly back.

Suddenly he fell back on the tried and tested tactic of finishing off his rival with some new revelation. 'I really didn't want to hurt you with this, but you know, you've got a completely wrong picture of Levin. On Christmas Eve, I went to see my brother in the Palatinate. The things I heard there . . .'

I flushed. This was beginning to sound ominous.

'Make it quick,' I said.

'Levin was having it off with Margot,' he said in a flat voice, and he watched me expectantly.

I came within an inch of giving myself away with a knowing nod.

'Not just then, when I was doing time,' Dieter went on. 'Probably here too, here in this house, when I was out with the truck and you were at work.'

So where did Dieter's brother get hold of such intimate details?

'She had started messing about with Klaus as well.'

A vague memory stirred in me. Long ago, Levin had told me something about Margot cheating on her husband with his best friend and his own brother. 'Was Margot's baby yours?' I asked.

'The kid? How was anybody supposed to know exactly? It's just as well I've only now found out about the business with Levin, or else I would have chucked her out of the window myself.'

At that, I went red a second time, and he noticed it. 'Hella . . . ?' he said, vaguely suspicious.

I burst into tears and made a show of pressing my hands

against my stomach. You had to treat pregnant women with care.

Dieter started rushing up and down. 'You're not . . . Are you . . . ?' he said, putting an arm round my shoulders.

I tried to shake my head.

He raised my chin and looked straight into my reddened eyes. 'Levin doesn't deserve your sympathy,' he said. 'He never showed any consideration for you.'

That was true enough. But it didn't stop me preaching. 'You don't pay like with like. I am going to talk to him, but when I think the time is right.'

'If a bad tooth has to come out,' Dieter countered, 'there's little point in putting things off.'

'Oh, but there is,' I said firmly. 'If the patient has an infection and a fever, you have to wait.' The next day, I went to see the sick child. Although her face was still spotty, Lene was by no means confined to bed, but was instead fighting with her brother over a new swing that had been fixed to a door frame. Pavel was happy to see me, as was Lene with the big parcel of Lego I had brought. Since the children called me by my first name, he and I went over to the same basis.

My cake was delicious, but I wanted to stay only a quarter of an hour, just for the tasting. While Pavel cleared the table, I read the children a story. The time just flew past, much too quickly. After I had finished reading, I looked into Pavel's honest face and I was overcome by a desire to be taken into his arms and to try out his grey-flecked whiskers against my cheek. 'We missed out on each other,' I thought, 'but at least we can become friends.'

The children switched on the television, so we kept our voices down as we chatted. After the birth of Lene, I found out, his wife fell ill, started hearing voices and inflicting injuries on herself. It had almost broken his heart when she had to be taken away from her children. There were periods, every now and then, when she was allowed home, but then she had to be heavily medicated.

'It may sound very cruel,' he said, 'but I'm almost glad when she has to go away again. The tension is too much for me, as well as the worry about the children's well-being.'

He took my hand. Without more than a moment's thought, I invited him over to our New Year's Eve party.

'I'd rather not,' said Pavel. 'When all that banging and crashing of the fireworks starts up, I wouldn't want to leave the children on their own. Quite apart from the fact that they still haven't really got over their illness.'

I had to agree. But my face must have taken on a worried expression. If the children were fast asleep around midnight, he said, giving way a little, then he might yet manage to come round. Otherwise he'd probably sit around feeling morose and shut in. But would it be all right by me if he didn't turn up until the party was almost over?

'You do just what you fancy, you don't have to tie yourself down at all,' I said. 'It's supposed to be no more than a cosy get-together, a few friends, some nice music and something good to eat.'

'Right, that's exactly the way I like it best,' said Pavel, and I took my leave.

On the morning of the thirty-first of December, Dorit called off. Now her children had caught measles. 'Oh, Lord,' I said, 'and now I've invited Pavel Siebert! But he probably won't be able to come either anyway. Have you ever seen his sick wife?'

'Yes, sure. There was a time when she was a raving beauty, but now! Listless, terribly listless. She's on some kind of sedative or other, looks all puffy. She came once to pick Lene up from kindergarten; it was a tragic sight! That lively, active child taking the hand of an absolute llama!'

Ever since our student days, Dorit and I had applied that term to lethargic people and, since we ourselves were the exact opposite of that, we tended rather to look down on them. I'm sure I must be a great deal more attractive to Pavel than a sick llama, I thought, but I've never been a raving beauty.

In the meantime, Levin had pulled himself together again, to

149

some extent. Sad-eyed, he would prowl around me like some motherless kitten, but at least he wasn't crying so much any more. Soon I'd have to have a serious talk with him. But what was I to say? 'Neither of you exactly fits the bill,' I thought, 'but the last thing I want is a fatherless child.'

Since Dorit and Gero weren't coming, I had bought far too much stuff. I hardly expected Pavel to come, since it didn't make much sense driving from Heidelberg to Viernheim at dead of night.

Dieter came into the kitchen. 'What goodies have we today?' he asked.

'Roast beef, nice and pink.'

'You mean bleeding,' said Dieter. 'Not for me, thanks, I get sick at the very sight of raw meat.'

Too bad about the expensive piece of loin; it simply tasted so much better when it hadn't been cooked right through. 'But Levin prefers it underdone,' I said, without really knowing whether he did or not.

Dieter's face darkened. 'Well of course the poor orphan is much more important, and anyway, I can always go down to the local.'

Anything but that. That would mean there was even more left over. 'No problem,' I said. 'I'll just leave your share ten minutes longer under the grill.'

Dieter was pacified. As good as gold, he peeled the potatoes for the gratin and cut them into thin slices.

Then Levin came into the kitchen with fresh peaches. 'From faraway lands. The afters are on me: fruit salad, with melon, peaches and black grapes.' While Levin always claimed he couldn't cook, he nevertheless always shopped for the ingredients for his favourite dishes. I had a look at the peaches. They were so hard you couldn't even get the skin off them.

16

'I just don't understand how anyone can so consistently come up with such duds,' said Rosemarie Hirte. 'But then, who am I to cast the first stone!'

'Go ahead, speak your mind,' I offered. 'Would you have plumped for Levin or for Dieter?'

She wrinkled her nose. A muttered 'I'd have made good Injuns of the pair of them,' I didn't quite catch, but a second comment followed after a while: 'Rich or poor, death is the great leveller.'

That day, she dedicated her whole attention to solving crossword puzzles, only occasionally asking for the name of a river in the Hindu Kush or some other thing that was all Greek to me. Only when I was able to supply 'gate-crasher' for 'uninvited guest' was she reminded of the New Year's party I had arranged.

Out of crushed garlic, mustard, olive oil, salt, freshly ground pepper and tomato purée, I concocted an emulsion-like paste. I cut the roast in half and speared the heavy grilling spit through both pieces. Carefully, I brushed the oily seasoning over the meat, cut onions into fine rings, laid them in the drip-tray and at last turned on the oven. The roast beef was rotating rather unevenly, but I knew from experience that it always turned out well in the end. Dieter had spread out the thinly sliced potatoes in a shallow casserole. Now he sprinkled them with salt and rosemary and poured cream over the lot. Levin was struggling away with his peaches.

The atmosphere of bustling activity in the warm kitchen gave rise once again to something like a cosy intimacy, the sort of thing we had enjoyed together in earlier days. Levin put on a record of hits from the thirties and even attempted a little

151

tap-dance. To 'Yes, we have no Bananas', he slipped on a piece of bacon rind that Dieter had used to grease the casserole.

'Sorry,' said Dieter contritely, 'it slipped out of my hand.'

Levin took it in good part. I was amazed at how placid he was.

Three-quarters of an hour later, I took one half of the roast out of the oven, wrapped it tightly in aluminium foil and put it aside to keep warm. Dieter's portion had to go on rotating for another fifteen minutes.

At last, we were sat at the beautifully-laid table in the conservatory, and then we noticed it was already eleven o'clock. 'Just right,' said Dieter. 'That means we can eat our way into the New Year, and that's as good a trick as any for warding off evil spirits.'

The meal looked terrific, and both Levin and Dieter were delighted with the bloody or unbloody condition of their respective pieces of meat. Even I had worked up an appetite, although the rich aromas still didn't agree with me and, after the smell of fat in the kitchen, I was glad to be back out in the conservatory.

Levin took the knife and fork from my hands. 'Duty of the master of the house,' he said. 'Even my grandad, the old patriarch, took it on himself to carve the meat.'

At once, he gave a disapproving shake of the head; the knife was too blunt for his liking. Ever since his unfinished training in dentistry, Levin had become used to precision instruments. He went to get the steel, which he handled with professional skill. 'Roast beef has to be cut paper-thin,' he pontificated.

As for me, I was just happy to see him with something to do.

Levin began with our underdone piece, expertly cutting off the first slice, which he laid on my plate.

Dieter, feeling queasy, averted his gaze as red juice flowed over the serving dish, on which his well-done piece of meat also lay. 'Bunch of cannibals,' he said.

Then we started eating, praising each other for our excellent cooking, raised our glasses all round and tried to play down any animosities that threatened to surface.

'Oh, look outside!' I exclaimed. 'It's snowing.'

What we had been denied at Christmas, the New Year was now about to bring us. From the jungle of the conservatory, and in the light shining out from it into the garden, we looked out into the white flakes steadily, incessantly swirling down to the ground.

Levin, always the big child, was delighted. 'It's a symbol,' he said. 'The New Year is starting as innocent as a newborn baby, wrapped in snow-white nappies. Everything on earth that's dirty is being covered up.'

'What half-baked claptrap,' said Dieter.

We both stared at him in alarm.

'If the coming year is supposed to represent a new beginning,' grumbled Dieter, 'then now's the time, shortly before twelve, to start with a clean sheet!'

Did he mean me?

Levin played all innocent. 'I'll clear away the dirty table cloth in good time, but first there's my delicious sweet. After that, we'll have a clean sheet.'

No one so much as smiled.

I tried to get hold of Dieter's hand under the table, but he snatched it violently away from me. 'You know exactly what I mean,' he said.

'No idea,' said Levin, uncertainly.

I was getting worried, so I started gathering up the plates.

'Hold on,' said Levin. 'I was just going to have one more piece of roast on its own!' He picked up the sharp knife.

Dieter went on undeterred. 'You were having it off with Margot.'

No reply. Levin tried to carry on as if concentrating on carving off a wafer-thin slice of meat, but his delicate hands were trembling.

'I'm waiting for an answer, if you don't mind,' bawled Dieter.

Levin stopped slicing and, with the large serving fork, put a tiny piece of meat in his mouth. I couldn't help thinking of Margot and 'Porky', the butcher. 'What do you want me to do?' he asked.

'I want you to admit it . . .' said Dieter.

'What?' Levin was stalling.

'I've heard all about it from my brother.'

Levin shrugged. 'We all know what Margot was like,' he said. 'It was her that wanted it, not me.'

True as that might be, Dieter still went on, menacingly, 'And now item two: you're going to have to get a divorce.'

It was only now that I got panicky, for I had been able to keep out of the row so far.

Levin was incensed. What did Dieter think he was talking about – after all, we were expecting a child, and Dieter should think himself lucky that I had listened to these tasteless accusations without going off into a fit of hysterics.

'The baby's mine,' said Dieter. 'The one that went wrong was very likely yours. So we're quits if you give Hella up to me.'

The knife dropped from Levin's hand. He was looking for an outright denial from me. I was trembling with fear. The last thing I wanted was to be passed on to this raving mad Dieter, as a substitute for Margot, as it were. I burst out crying for all I was worth, anything to prevent an inquisition.

'You're out of your mind,' said Levin, plucking up his courage. 'The baby's mine, one hundred per cent. Well, go on, Hella, tell him!'

'Whenever Hella tells you the truth, you always put on that hurt and humiliated act,' said Dieter. 'She wanted to spare you after your mother died, or else she would have let the cat out of the bag long ago!'

Levin shook me as if I were that bag. 'Well, say something, can't you? Tell him he's off his head!'

But he couldn't even shake a single word of sense out of me.

'Just sod off, you bastard!' shouted Levin, his voice filled with venom. 'All you've ever done is bring trouble into my house! Get back to the gutter where you belong!'

Dieter swung his fist. With one powerful blow, he felled my tall, but delicate, husband. Blood spurted from Levin's mouth, and the sight of it made Dieter feel sick. I made towards the telephone to call the police.

When Levin gasped out 'Hospital!' in between spitting blood and teeth, all I called for was an ambulance.

Dieter was puking into my stainless steel sink, and didn't emerge from the kitchen again.

From the bathroom, I brought warm water and towels. Levin was moaning loudly. At that very moment, the bells started ringing in the New Year.

I was sitting on the floor, holding up Levin's head to stop him swallowing blood, and trying to staunch the flow by pressing damp towels on it. Thankfully, I soon heard the ambulance's siren outside.

Green about the gills, Dieter came back on the scene. 'They're here,' he said. 'I'm off. On no account must you tell them how it happened!'

I protested. 'I've got to tell the truth . . .'

'You should have thought of that sooner,' said Dieter. 'Tell them Levin slipped on that piece of bacon rind and smashed his face open on the cooker.'

With that, he slunk, coatless, out through the conservatory door and disappeared into the swirling snow. I had to leave Levin to let the ambulance-men in. On my way to the front door, I made a hasty detour by way of the kitchen to hide Dieter's cutlery and plate in the larder.

The ambulance crew didn't waste a moment, but put on a temporary dressing and lifted Levin on to a stretcher. Despite their haste, they still wanted to know how it had happened.

'An accident,' I said, following orders. 'He slipped and hit his head on the cooker.'

One of the men gave me a hard look. 'So why's he not lying in the kitchen?' he demanded.

'He . . . he managed to stagger this far before he went down,' I assured them. 'I've already mopped up the trail of blood.'

'Typical housewife,' said the ambulance-man. 'The man's practically bleeding to death and the first thing the wife does is wipe the floor!'

I couldn't get the picture of Levin's chalk-white, blood-smeared face out of my head. How small that face was,

155

and how enormous Dieter's fist had been. In an attempt to take my mind off it, I set to work on the floor, cleared the table, put the fruit salad in the fridge and disposed of the leftovers.

Once I had the kitchen and the conservatory in some sort of order again, I ran a full bath, laced it with a relaxing essence and climbed into the warm water.

At long last I was able to think straight. 'The main thing is, my baby's fine,' I thought, not without a degree of defiance.

Finally, I put on my nightdress and dressing-gown and went back out to the conservatory. Tamerlane had disappeared; no doubt animals suffered when their masters were bashing each other's heads in.

'Ta – mer – lane,' I called out into the garden in my most soothing voice. Through the gently falling snowflakes, the cat appeared and came warily closer. 'Hey-ho, hey-ho, Pussy's in the snow,' I sang, feeling as if I should have been playing in a film.

With the cat in my arms, I lay down in the hammock, shivering despite my hot bath. I could neither think clearly nor fall asleep, and the night was still far from over.

At half past one, the phone rang. Dorit, of course, I thought, ringing up to wish me a Happy New Year. That was more than I could take. But when it went on ringing, I finally did drag myself to the phone. It was bound to be the hospital, and Levin was dead.

It was in fact the clinic, but Levin was recovering. They had stopped the nosebleed and stitched his burst upper lip. Still, he was now short of his four top front teeth. If they could be brought in right away, they could preserve them and later on an attempt to re-implant them could be made in the Dental Hospital at Heidelberg University.

I had found one tooth and already consigned it to the waste-bin. I presumed the others would be outside in the snow, because, on his way to hospital, Levin had been spitting copiously.

'They're lying under a covering of snow,' I said wearily. 'Tomorrow, when it's light, I can have a good look for them.'

They reckoned that would probably be too late. Exhausted as I was, I was just staggering back into my hammock when suddenly a huge icicle appeared before me. Like the cat before him, Dieter had sneaked back in from the darkness of the garden.

'Hella, it's all *your* fault!' he said, reproachfully. The enormity of this accusation set me off in a rage.

'Was *I* the one who made Levin a hospital case?' I screamed.

'If you had come straight out and told him I'm the father, none of this would have happened. You're a coward.'

Tamerlane, my furry hot-water bottle, leapt from my lap. On the smooth tiled floor, he started swiping a tiny object around in all directions, as if life was all of a sudden just one big game.

'What's that he's got?' I asked, to change the subject.

Dieter had a look. It was a tooth. 'How's Levin?' he asked.

'You've knocked out his front teeth.'

Dieter appeared to have no regrets. 'Serves him right. The time for going easy on him is past.'

'Oh, Dieter,' I said, so worn out I wasn't thinking. 'Maybe he is the father after all. How am I supposed to know exactly?'

Dieter froze. 'Say that again!'

Like some lioness, I roared, 'For God's sake, leave me in peace! I don't know. It's probably neither of you lousy bastards!'

Everything happened so quickly I can't reconstruct it any more. I was lying on the floor, having been roughly hauled out of the hammock, Dieter had thrown himself on top of me and was trying to throttle me.

'Whore!' he was yelling over and over.

All my struggling and thrashing about was to no avail; he was as strong as an ox. I'll never forget the mortal fear I felt then. But in the end I lapsed into a kind of faint and all fear left me. I became completely calm. Swathed in clouds and mist, I saw Pavel as God the Father, with his bushy beard. And then, suddenly, I could breathe again. The grip on my throat relaxed and the weight on top of me lifted.

Dazed, I sat up. Nearby, Pavel and Dieter were wrestling on the floor.

If only the police were there! I tried to get to my feet. Pavel's face was turning blue and he was struggling for air. Dieter was bawling, 'So this is the great stud that sneaks into the house at night and knocks you up!'

I had to do something, and fast. I thumped a ceramic pot with a yellow cock's comb on it down on Dieter's back – without the slightest effect. But what was that glinting next to me in the earthenware pot of one of the philodendrons? The sharp carving knife that Levin had dropped.

While I'm a clever chemist and a good housewife, and I'm stronger than people think, I'm a dead loss at knife-throwing. It flew low through the air and missed Dieter's back completely, only grazing his arm. Obviously he felt no more than a slight jab, but it was enough to take his attention off Pavel and make him look round. The sight of drops of his own blood made him feel faint again.

Pavel managed to get his right hand free from under Dieter's weight and to grab the knife. But before he could do any more than get a grip of it, Dieter passed out and fell on the blade.

Once Pavel had got shakily to his feet, he was in command, shouting, 'The police!' I rushed to the phone.

I was quivering when I got back into the conservatory, and Pavel took me in his arms. Like Hansel and Gretel, we stood there, clinging dumbly to each other and repeatedly stroking each other's back for consolation. Neither of us dared so much as to glance at the badly injured man.

When the police and ambulance arrived, we were still in no fit state to be questioned. I was given a sedative injection. Pavel refused.

The ambulance-men, the same ones who had already carted Levin off, were vital witnesses to the fact that an incident had occurred in this house earlier on; unfortunately, though, that made matters worse for us, if anything, since I hadn't told the truth about Levin's injuries.

After the police had taken photographs and done a forensic

investigation of the conservatory, Pavel and I had to go along with them to the station to sign statements. Then, at the hospital, our bruises from the attempted strangulation were examined and recorded by a doctor.

At long last, we were allowed to go. I begged Pavel to stay with me, because the last thing I wanted was to be left on my own. But that wasn't possible – he was already suffering pangs of conscience on account of his children.

'I'll phone you in the morning,' he promised. 'And then we'll take it from there.'

In an attempt to calm myself down, I spent the rest of the night watering my plants in the conservatory. The dwarf coconut palm and the prickly Christ's-thorn seldom required water, whereas the specimens from Guyana needed plenty of warmth and humidity, and the South American spotted fern got my full attention with the watering can. My poor conservatory, so often desecrated already, was going to receive all the love and care I was capable of; but both Tamerlane and the orchids seemed to be staring at me in pained reproach.

17

'New Year's Eve snow ne'er did make riches grow,' sneered my room-mate.

I hate stupid sayings, if that was what she was supposed to have come out with, so I shot back, 'There's no fool like an old fool.'

She took no offence. 'Some perfume?' she asked.

Was she trying to tell me I smelled? 'Do we have consultant's rounds tonight?' I asked, since she was spraying it on particularly thick.

But the heart-throb didn't come. Instead, it was Dr Kaiser. We were sour at him because lately he had stopped us having any coffee. The night sister had blabbed to him that we were chattering so much at night we never got any sleep. Once again, he cut my queries stone dead – he knew perfectly well what was good for me.

'It may have slipped your memory that I'm a qualified chemist,' I said with all the arrogance I could muster.

Gerhard Kaiser is one of those who back down easily.

Rosemarie seemed to be observing his capitulation with some relish.

Later, she thought of something else: 'Snow and ice on New Year's Day bring only trouble and strife your way . . .'

'Right for once,' I said. 'Who would fancy shovelling snow after a sleepless night! But I had to, since there wasn't a man around.'

Once I had fulfilled this arduous civic duty with shovel and broom, I decided to crawl back to bed with Tamerlane. I had put the phone away well out of earshot, to protect myself from my family's good wishes. Nor did I want to be kept in touch as to Dieter's and Levin's condition.

There are a few refuges in human life which everyone

uses when things are going badly: me, I put bed top of the list. Whenever I'm up to my ears in troubles, then that's the one and only panacea. I admit, I was often tempted to bring on sleep by artificial means – heaven knows there was never any lack of medical preparations about the house. Dorit can't lay down her head without Valium, and her example always served as a warning to me. Most of the time, I've managed to conquer my insomnia with tea, valerian and similar harmless household remedies.

Sleep and death are brothers, they say. And so my fondness for bed is probably not a very positive attitude, but it does bring a kind of healing of the mind. Besides, if you just lie there long enough, new life-forces usually awake.

There were a thousand things I had to take in hand. If it came to a divorce, Levin would want to lay down certain financial conditions. As far as I was concerned, he could grab part of the shares and bonds for himself if he wanted; half of the money along with the villa would be quite enough for me. Should I perhaps set up in business for myself? I could live with my child in the upstairs rooms and fit out a chemist's shop on the ground floor. Would I be able to afford a nanny? No doubt my parents would go off their heads again about my new lifestyle.

As always happened, I found this planning cheered me up no end. Of course, I couldn't very well torment Levin with my plans for divorce, not right away. To start a row with him, when he was missing his four front teeth, would be unfair. All the same, a sense that there was some providential justice about it all kept making me grin to myself; his third set of teeth would always be there to remind him of a certain glass dish.

Now that he had almost succeeded in strangling me, I didn't give Dieter a second thought. Well, yes, he wasn't a completely worthless character when you came down to it, and in other circumstances . . . I had to concede that it had in fact been his colourful past that had attracted me.

Now, however, there was suddenly a third man on the scene, Pavel. A sweet soul, the kind of man you occasionally had to polish his glasses for, or pick the odd bit of dried-up egg yolk out of his beard. What sort of chance did I have there? Up till now, I had the impression that Pavel liked me all right, but that he was sticking by the mother of his children.

When, in the afternoon, hunger drove me from my bed, I simply ignored the ringing phone. I made some tea and stuffed cold roast beef into my mouth. The more I ate, the greedier I got, and Tamerlane, too, couldn't seem to satisfy his appetite on his usual cat-food. We shared a tin of tuna. I mashed my half and mixed in capers, ketchup, raw onions and lemon juice.

That evening, the door-bell rang. I slipped to the window and sneaked a look out. Pavel was shocked at the sight of me – I suppose I must have looked pretty wan.

'Are you ill?' he said on seeing I was still in a housecoat.

'Maybe a little. I'm still suffering from the shock.'

'And how is our strangler getting on?' he asked.

I shrugged. 'Maybe he's died in the meantime,' I said.

Pavel's eyebrows went up in surprise. He phoned the hospital, to hear that only close relatives would be given information on Dieter's state of health. But then, I knew that ever since Margot's accident.

'But I suppose I have to conclude from that that he's still in the land of the living,' said Pavel. 'And how's your husband?'

I assured Pavel (although he didn't catch my drift) that Levin had been my husband long enough and that I had no desire to go and visit him now.

'It's too late anyway,' said Pavel. 'In hospitals, the evening meal is served at five and lights-out is at eight, which is why they're wakened at six. But we could still phone the ward.'

I didn't want to.

We sat drinking tea together. 'Where have you left your children?' I asked.

'A neighbour's sitting with them, reading to them from *Heidi*,' he said, and I felt a little twinge. 'A pretty, young neighbour?' I asked, my attempt at irony failing miserably.

Pavel merely grinned.

Still, he had been worried about me, only as a single parent he didn't have much spare time and had to leave again soon. All the same, I felt fortified, because there was a positive aura about Pavel, the kind of thing I had missed in my previous men-friends.

The next day, I felt strong enough to go and see Levin in hospital. He was lying in a ward with two beds. At first, all I could see was this weird profile that looked remarkably like an ant-eater's. The area all round Levin's mouth and nose had been stitched and bandaged, and was swollen and suffused with purple. He couldn't talk and was making painful efforts to suck on a straw jutting sideways out of his proboscis.

'How's it going?' I asked, a totally superfluous question.

He rolled his eyes despairingly heavenwards.

'Well, in this sort of situation, I suppose you just have to grit your teeth,' I said with malicious cheerfulness.

Then I sat with him for a while and became a little more chatty. Did he want me to tell him the next chapter about Dieter's running amok? Levin indicated that he knew all about it. He wrote on a notepad that a policeman had come to question him, but had realized that Levin was in no fit condition to make a statement. Nevertheless, he had let slip that Dieter had been severely injured and was in the same hospital, in intensive care.

'Will he pull through?' I asked.

Levin didn't know.

I showed my bruises from the attempted throttling, and he nodded his appreciation. We were partners in suffering. We broached neither the paternity question nor the subject of divorce.

'Is there something I can bring you? Books, fruit juice, custard?' I asked.

Levin wrote out, 'Travel books, comics, nothing sour to drink, maybe banana juice.'

I promised I would.

Then I took myself off to the area outside the intensive care ward. The ward sister was making no predictions, telling me

163

only that no one who had just come through an operation could be allowed visitors.

I was no sooner back home than I phoned Pavel. 'Should we come over to you, or will you come here?' he asked.

The children felt at their ease at my place, and fortunately I always had plenty of milk and drinking chocolate handy, as well, because of the season of the year, as mountains of Christmas cakes and biscuits.

With the help of their father, little Lene and her brother Kolya built a snowman, round which Tamerlane stalked suspiciously. 'Do you have a sledge?' Kolya asked.

I did have one, but unfortunately no suitable hill on the premises to go with it.

That gave Pavel the idea of driving off into the mountains with the children for a few days. 'Would you like to come?' he asked.

I could think of nothing I'd like more, but the prospect of a long drive to Switzerland or Austria filled me with horror.

'There's no need for that at all,' Pavel said. 'I'm not exactly your keen sporty type. For me, it would be enough just to go tobogganing with the children, and we can do that in the Odenwald. It would do the two of them a world of good after their measles.'

We hesitated no longer, for the school holidays were already nearing their end.

Pavel drove us to a small spa in the hills. In the car park, the snow was by now far from gleaming white, with exhaust fumes having left their mark like cinnamon on the sugary powdered snow, while the scarred earth looked like grated chocolate. All eager for action, we tumbled out, then stopped at once to admire the distant views. Over towards the horizon, the mountains were brighter, their wintry colours even softer, as one range of hills rose behind the other, like a series of arches. Grey apple trees stood embedded in white fields, enriching the palette of the winter landscape alongside the green of the bramble bushes and the reddish browns of the

164

beech leaves. Here, dark firs, black crows, and over there, the wall of a churchyard.

We went walking along gentle hilltops, crept through cattle fences, let the children climb up into hunting hides and do tightrope walks along fallen tree trunks, and in a moss-covered shelter we shared out jelly-babies. To his uninterested son, Pavel explained how you could recognize the points of the compass by looking for the greener, weather side of trees, examined a display panel showing indigenous species of songbirds and joined his children in hacking cracks into the layer of ice on frozen puddles with the heel of his boot. A jay followed us as we went.

When I looked back, my heart warmed to the sight of all our various footprints in the snow – an expert tracker would have recognized the signs of a happy little family.

Towards the end of our long walk, the children, too lazy to continue, let themselves be pulled along on the sledge. Then finally, we settled in a warm hostelry and played 'I spy with my little eye'.

Once all the green, red and who knows how many other coloured objects had been guessed, Pavel claimed he could see something golden.

We tried and tried, and couldn't get it.

'It's Hella's heart,' he said, and the kids protested that that didn't count.

My heart of gold was beating hard.

Rosemarie Hirte grumbled, 'Since when! Golden! Don't make me laugh! But then of course you're a sucker for such sentimental tosh!'

'Which of you,' Pavel asked his children at last, 'wants to sleep in my room, and which in Hella's?'

I had feared something like this would happen.

The children looked at me and maintained a tactful silence. Then Lene said, 'I want to go with my daddy.'

For all that he was only six, Kolya was already far too polite to reject my company outright. 'The best thing would be if the grown-ups sleep in one room and the children in the other.'

Pavel and I looked at each other. I nodded, perhaps a little too hastily.

Well, we did sleep in one and the same room, but not with each other. We lay chatting for ages like some close married couple, then Pavel switched off the light. In the middle of the night, I could sense a visitor to my bed; it was Lene. I turned on the bedside lamp and could see Kolya lying beside his father.

I had sent word to Levin that I was going away for a few days. No doubt he took that amiss, but I wanted to do my unborn child a favour. The three days in the snow, the long walks and afternoon naps did me a power of good, too.

When, after my first day back at work, I sat at Levin's bedside again, he was already able to mumble his reproaches. He didn't ask where I had been, merely bemoaned his own toothless existence. He was to be allowed home in two days' time, but then he faced the whole rigmarole at the dentist's.

'And what about Dieter?' I asked.

Strangely enough, Levin had been to pay him a visit. Dieter was no longer in the intensive care ward and was on the way to recovery, but he was in a state of utter depression. Having it all out with the pair of them was out of the question.

When Levin was discharged, I couldn't very well send him packing straight away; I had by this time shifted his bed into the little study anyway. A few days later, he raised, as was only to be expected, the question as to who was the real father of the baby.

I couldn't come up with any judgement of Solomon. I admitted I had slept with Dieter. But since he and Margot had . . . 'The best thing would be for us to get a divorce right away.'

For days on end, Levin didn't bring up the subject again, but seemed deep in thought.

Each afternoon, after closing time, I went to visit my new friend. We would embrace warmly, but there was never

166

more in it than that. The children were beginning to grow attached to me.

I owe many musical experiences to men-friends. One of them introduced me to Mozart, another to Satchmo. Levin was fond of old hits and the Beatles. Pavel had a piano and would sing children's songs with Lene. He had a gorgeous baritone voice. Sometimes he would put on a little concert for me, singing Mahler or Brahms, then he would become embarrassed and break off in roars of laughter whenever he sang or played a wrong note.

I was enchanted.

One day, he showed me old photographs of his wife. 'Pretty as a picture,' or something like that, was what Dorit had called her. But when you knew of her madness, it was already there to be seen. I felt a shiver down my back, as if this figure had arisen out of another world.

'Lovely,' I said, tactfully.

'Beautiful, but dishonest,' said Pavel. 'The first signs of her illness occurred while she was still in her adolescence, but she kept that from me. Well, I suppose anyone might have done the same.'

We trusted each other. Pavel became the first and only outsider to get to hear about my problem with the two fathers. I was grateful to him that he didn't laugh.

One day, I found him, too, in a bad mood. Without a word, he held out a letter he had received by recorded delivery: his landlady had given him notice to quit. 'Now I've got to start house-hunting all over again,' said Pavel. 'God, how I hate that! If you hear of anywhere that's on the market, do let me know.'

Working in a chemist's, you do in fact hear a lot, most especially about people who have died. But the last thing Pavel wanted was to go running to the relatives of someone recently deceased to ask if he could have the flat that had fallen vacant.

For days, I pondered the matter. I wanted so much to live under the same roof as Pavel. There was plenty of room in my house, but how were we to share out the rooms? Just as I was about to make Pavel the offer, Dieter was discharged from hospital. He still needed looking after, naturally, but the course of medical treatment had been completed.

I would probably have refused delivery of this piece of goods, but Levin had already welcomed Dieter and paid off his taxi. Now he lay convalescing in his bedroom, and Levin, with gritted teeth, was taking a meal up to him. So we seemed to be back where we started.

I went up the stairs in a rage. I hadn't seen Dieter since that fateful New Year's Eve. Now four weeks had slipped by and, while the dark bruises on my throat had disappeared, my mental scars had not.

Dieter was pale, had lost a lot of weight, and seemed desperately miserable. He looked at me like someone at death's door. I couldn't bring myself either to throw him out into the street or to heap reproaches on his head. With great ill-humour, I just had to accept his presence.

The next day, I described my predicament to Pavel, the two would-be fathers of my child at home again, both of them ailing, and both in a lousy frame of mind.

'So how do they get on together?' Pavel asked. 'I mean, they must detest each other.'

That was very probably so, yet for all that, they weren't gouging each other's eyes out, but providing mutual support in their pain and suffering.

'And which one of them now believes himself to be the true procreator?' asked Pavel, bewildered.

'Both of them. But I hereby declare you to be the father of my choice and deny them both the right to paternity on the grounds of their undesirable conduct.'

Pavel laughed.

18

'Your old Pavel could at least smuggle in a jar of Nescafé with him,' said Rosemarie. 'After all, he gets plenty of butter from us.'

'But what about hot water?'

'I'll get that from the ward kitchen. All we'd need then would be a thermos flask.'

I nodded. All just a question of organization.

At that, the consultant suddenly came in, without his usual train. Rosemarie beamed at him, even though she had had no chance either to spray herself with perfume or put on a fresh nightdress for him.

He was bringing her good news: the latest test results were just in, no sign of cancer cells.

'I knew that,' she said.

'Tomorrow we're going to take out your catheter, and you can go home at the weekend,' he said.

I was speechless.

'And your time's getting close, too,' he said to me. 'And then we'll have to transfer you to Ward II . . .'

So we were soon to be parted.

That afternoon, Dorit found me in tears.

'Your boss is refusing to give me any more Valium without a prescription. What on earth am I going to do?' she complained.

On Tuesday afternoons, Ortrud was always on her own in the shop; I scribbled a note – with only a hint of blackmail in it – to my former colleague.

'Why can't she just get the stuff from her doctor?' Rosemarie demanded naively.

'Oh, what do they know about anything?' I said. 'Heartless lot.'

* * *

169

After the traumatic events of New Year's Eve, Dorit had phoned several times, and I had had to keep putting her off. I would make excuses like the soup was just boiling over, or I was dead tired, the door-bell had just rung that very moment, or I was expecting a call from my boss. Dorit began to smell a rat and demanded my presence. 'No lame excuses,' she said.

She knew far too much already. Lene had been playing with Dorit's daughter and had let slip that I went to visit them daily. Like some strait-laced governess, Dorit demanded an explanation.

'We're fond of each other,' I said, as off-hand as I could, 'but if you start thinking you can sniff scandal, you're on the wrong track.'

'Not in the least. You are pregnant, don't forget,' she assured me. 'Anyone knows that children of that age often get carried away by their imagination. Lene was prattling on about you having shared a room with Pavel – in a hotel – and the children had both been there too. You see through that right away: wishful thinking on the part of a motherless child . . .'

We exchanged searching looks.

'So what does Levin have to say about your friendship?' she asked.

'He was in the hospital at the time,' I said, although I realized that wasn't exactly the right answer.

But it was enough to divert her attention. 'What's wrong with him then?' she inquired sympathetically.

'Dieter knocked out his four front teeth.'

Dorit gaped at me, incredulous. 'Why?'

'Drunk,' I said.

She stared in horror. 'I just hope you kicked that Dieter out on the spot, but then I'm afraid you're just daft enough . . .'

She talked to me as if I were sick. All right, I wasn't exactly a redeeming angel, but certainly too good for that dreadful company. She would have to have a word with Levin, to make sure he got rid of Dieter, and right away.

For the first time in our long-standing friendship, we got into a real row. She accused me of being simple-minded and having a thing about social responsibilities.

In the end, I spat it out: 'It could be that the baby's Dieter's!'

Dorit refused to believe me. I was, she said, beyond all redemption.

Once Dieter was feeling better, I summoned Levin to a sickbed conference. Levin was wearing false teeth, which he detested; his fury was concentrated on me, rather than on the aggressor responsible for them.

'She's going to make us draw lots for the baby,' said Levin.

Dieter gave me a woebegone look.

Next thing, we'll have the two of them blubbing all over the place, I thought. 'No,' I said, 'but what I do want is for you both to find somewhere else to stay. I don't want to live together with you any longer.'

'What have we done to deserve that?' whined Levin.

'Dieter has nearly killed me, and you two-timed me with Margot right from the very start.'

'Well, yes, all right, so now we're quits,' said Levin.

Dieter, who hardly said a word at all these days, spoke up at last. 'If you two throw me out on the street now, I'll do myself in,' he said, so grimly it was immediately credible.

'What do you mean by "you two",' said Levin. 'Me too, she wants me . . .'

'Okay,' I said, 'I'm not so heartless that you have to move into a shelter for the homeless this very day. But in future I want the ground floor for myself alone. You can move yourselves into the first floor together until you've found something suitable.'

Neither of them uttered another word.

The ground-floor flat had been cleared by the very next evening. In my absence, Levin had removed his goods and chattels upstairs, to settle in there in a cosy *ménage à deux* with Dieter.

When I made Pavel the offer to move in with me, he turned it down. 'You can't expect me to bring up my children right next to a madman . . . !' He broke off, suddenly thinking of his wife. 'I mean, a man prone to violence.'

Gradually, spring was approaching. It always arrived here in the Bergstrasse region first. In March, all the children gathered for the procession celebrating the first day of summertime, at which they burned an enormous cotton-wool snowman on the marketplace. In early April, my magnolia started blooming, but sadly the beautiful, pale pink blossoms turned brown under the incessant downpours and soon lay limp on the ground. When the cherry trees burst into huge white bouquets, I reckoned I could feel the baby's first movements. My pregnancy was going along excellently, and the gynaecologist was satisfied.

Despite Levin's mitigating evidence, Dieter was given a prison sentence, which he was to start very soon. Now and then, we would meet at the front door. He was thoroughly ashamed, which touched me a little. Sometimes I could feel him watching me from the first floor as I sat in the garden. I imagined he was having a good look at my bulging tummy, which was gradually rounding out.

Levin, too, kept well out of my way. At the start, I had been afraid the two of them might try to use the conservatory and, especially, the kitchen in my absence. But since they were both skilful do-it-yourselfers, they had put together a little cooking corner upstairs. I sneaked up to have a look at it for myself while they were out. You could hardly call it a provisional arrangement – a high-tech cooker, a hulking great fridge, double sink-unit with running water laid on, and several stainless steel cupboards had all been installed; all that was missing was tiles on the walls. They slept in separate rooms and it seemed to be more of a partnership of convenience than cohabitation.

Levin did inquire on two occasions as to the state of my health, but he made no demands whatsoever for either money or any other kind of service.

If I hadn't had at least a comradely relationship with Pavel, I might have felt a bit lonely. But against that, I was plagued by perpetual tiredness, I went to bed early and was only too glad that, after work and a visit to Pavel's, I didn't have to be there at anyone else's bidding.

One day, it finally came to the point where I felt so much in need of loving care that, after our welcoming embrace, I didn't want to let go of Pavel. 'What's the matter?' he asked anxiously.

I liked practically everything about this man. (The fact that he occasionally wore knee-breeches and insisted on a daily dose of listening to Schubert's *'Die schöne Müllerin'* was something I was sure I could wean him off in time.) I had an all-consuming desire to sleep with him, that's what the matter was. But apparently he was oblivious to that; sooner or later, I'd have to venture a direct attack.

Just as I was reluctantly releasing Pavel, Kolya approached, full of pompous self-importance, and informed me, 'Mummy's coming at the weekend.'

While I had always had to reckon with this possibility, I had usually managed to banish the thought from my mind. 'Are you looking forward to that?' I asked the boy.

He gave me an earnest look. 'No,' he said.

Then Lene piped up, 'You see, Mummy's ill.'

Pavel put me in the picture. This was a trial period, with his wife being allowed, for the time being, to spend the weekends at home in an attempt to accustom herself once more to a normal life.

'The children will tell her about me,' I said once Lene and Kolya were out of earshot.

'They did that long ago,' said Pavel.

My conscience pricked me. The woman must hate me. I was taking up some of her space here. 'How did she react?' I asked.

'Good heavens, she's much too ill to take an interest in any possible consequences of our friendship. She's only too grateful that you spend so much time with the children.'

I couldn't quite believe that, but it did come as something of a relief. After all, Pavel hadn't deceived his wife, much as I would have liked him to. He had probably told her how some happily married woman, expecting her own child, had struck up something of a friendship with their two.

'Do you think it would be wise for me to put in an appearance here at the weekend?' I asked.

Pavel shook his head. 'It's all a bit too much for her already.' He sounded depressed. 'Our having to move is going to be another big problem,' he said. 'Now I've got to tell her we can't stay here any longer.' His face was a picture of misery.

That lonely weekend, I went to see Dorit. She was angry with me because Dieter was still living upstairs. 'Just imagine the worst that could happen, and he throws another tantrum and chucks you down the stairs.'

'No, Dorit, deep down inside, he's really . . .'

Dorit just didn't understand me any more. 'I'm gradually coming to the conclusion that you should steer clear of men once and for all. You don't exactly have a lucky touch. Bring up your child on your own; it's no more than you deserve.'

'I could make a go of it with Pavel.'

'Pavel is married – and so are you.'

Where this sort of thing was concerned, Dorit's outlook was very old-fashioned, probably because she considered her own marriage to be the norm.

After my visit to Dorit's, I felt like taking a little stroll on my own; it was a mild, spring day, and I set off along a path by the River Neckar. I had steered practically all my previous lovers along here, for a kiss and cuddle by moonlight, and here I intended to walk proudly with my baby in its pram. The ducks, too, were taking their young for an outing, angry swans were stretching their already long necks because they had a nest hidden in the bushes to protect.

And a family of humans was coming towards me too: Pavel with his wife and the two children, who had spied me from a distance and now came running towards me. I was immediately on edge, for the last thing I wanted was for Pavel to imagine I had planned this chance meeting.

Alma held out her thin hand towards me; it felt like a dead mouse.

'The children have told me a lot about you,' she said politely.

Pavel was giving me a strange look. He was very uneasy.

Whenever I try to describe Alma's appearance, paintings come to my mind, either Art Nouveau or Romantic ones. Yes, it was true, she could have stepped out of a fairy story. The flowing silk dress was of an old-fashioned cut and emphasized to her advantage her anaemic complexion, her straw hat was decorated with pink ribbons (for all that, at that time of year, every ray of the sun was more than welcome), while her grey shoes had high heels (totally unsuitable there on the damp banks of the Neckar). All the colours she wore were soft, her voice was gentle and her eyes seemed clouded. 'All we need is for her to fall in a swoon,' I thought angrily. It was perfectly obvious this puffy-faced creature was in no state to clean a toilet.

'Come with us, Hella,' said Lene. 'That would be more fun. We're going to race each other.'

With all the dignity I could muster, I declined, saying my tummy would get in the way.

Alma was ghosting around in my dreams. Even in those few minutes, she had made a lasting impression on me. She certainly didn't look an invalid, either physically or, for that matter, mentally, but rather like some artful child dressing itself up as a grown woman. If I had come across Pavel ten years earlier, both of us could have been spared all manner of things, but what good was it going to do me to keep telling myself that?

Because of my advancing pregnancy, I was excused night duty. But at home, I had no help of any sort, and had to take out my own refuse, clean the stairs and windows in my flat and do my shopping. Only the garden was kept in order (presumably by Dieter). I took on a Portuguese woman, who came once a week to do the cleaning. What Levin did to fill his days, I had no idea; certainly, at night, the Porsche was frequently not in its usual place.

Pavel was able to find a suitable flat. Nevertheless, since it was safe to assume that Dieter was due to take up residence in a cell in the near future, he was still playing with the idea of moving in with me. I could sense that he was not altogether easy in his mind when he finally agreed – but only as an interim measure. He had decided to put most of his household goods in store.

Despite my swelling bay-window and my chronic tiredness, I helped him with the packing and removal. If Alma was coming for her usual visit at the weekend, there was to be no heavy work done that might upset her. I was beginning to envy the woman her quiet little corner.

On the day of the move, Dorit had come to fetch Pavel's children round to her place, while I took the day off to give the removal men their instructions as to which pieces of furniture belonged in which rooms. Pavel stood around meekly, getting in my way. Each of the children was given an attic room, while Pavel got the study.

Only that evening did I sense that I had been thoroughly overdoing things. I fell asleep on the sofa, dead to the world.

The next morning, I had to go to work, so any thought of a cosy breakfast without the children around was out of the question.

'So where did Alma get her old-fashioned clothes from?' asked Rosemarie, practical as ever.

'From rich parents with a bad conscience.'

'I get the feeling we're slowly approaching the happy end,' said Rosemarie, 'and not before time, either. I can't get the old phrase out of my head "Home sweet home".'

'Sweet it was, but only temporarily. We were on our own for the time being. Dieter was in jail, Levin was off on his travels. Except for the separate bedrooms, everything was just as I had dreamt it.'

19

'I know what would be a good name for the baby,' said Rosemarie Hirte.

Never mind that I had forbidden her to say a word about the problem in my womb. She was beginning to suspect that I was covering up my own fears by telling my story.

'But everything was all right at the last ultrasound scan, wasn't it?' she tried to calm me.

She would keep on trying to get round my ban on the subject. Naturally, thanks to Dr Kaiser's loose tongue, she had known all about it for some time: because of an anomaly in the placenta, the embryo was not receiving sufficient nourishment; my second child was too small for its age. Very soon, they were going to start inducing a premature delivery, because the baby would have a better chance of proper feeding once it was outside my body.

'So what name do you have in mind?'

Rosemarie smiled. 'What do you think of "Witold"?'

'But it's definitely going to be a girl. And anyway, we'd better wait until . . .'

'Okay, let's drop it. On with the family idyll!'

Pavel had been to see Alma in the hospital, and she was demanding to be allowed to spend another weekend with her children.

'That would be too much for me to ask of you,' grumbled Pavel.

Although I was none too keen on the idea of having Alma, difficult as she was, under my roof, I nevertheless said, big-hearted as ever, 'Why ever not, if she's so keen . . . ?'

By this time the days were getting warmer, things were

blooming in the garden. The children wanted to play outside; for the most part, Pavel would probably be able to keep Alma by his side out in the fresh air, so that I would have a little peace and quiet and would be able to take a lie down at regular intervals. I needed rest. But it was all to turn out differently.

I was sitting in the conservatory with the children, reading 'The Ugly Duckling' to them, Pavel having driven off to collect Alma. But barely five minutes later, Lene shouted, 'There's a car! Daddy's coming!'

We went to the window and saw Levin and a stranger unloading cases from the Porsche. Both of them tanned and in quite impractical white suits, looking like young gentlemen of the world for whom the exotic aromas of the wide-open spaces are like an underarm deodorant. On top of it all, they were both wearing weird sunglasses and jaunty hats, which certainly didn't suit Levin of all people. He had put on a pimpish grin, the like of which I had never seen on him. I heaved a sigh and drew the children back from the window, so as not to suggest to my husband that a fond welcome was awaiting him.

Later, Pavel and Alma arrived. Thankfully, the globe trotters didn't put in an appearance, but from upstairs came sounds of moving about and water running – no doubt they were unpacking and showering.

Pavel had got the message the moment he had seen the Porsche. Only behind Alma's back did he make inquiring gestures, pointing upwards. With a nod, I confirmed his suspicions.

Alma was obviously strained after her trip. She went straight to the hammock for a lie down and let the children rock her, with Tamerlane lying on top of her. The sight of this pretty picture filled me with disgust. Not only that, but I then had to serve Alma a laxative herbal tea by her hammock-side. Pavel begged me to suggest to her we got on first-name terms.

* * *

As we sat at table, there was a knock at the door, which immediately swung open. Levin and the newcomer traipsed in, with a casual 'Hello' all round, and then proceeded to stare pointedly at the steaming dumplings and the stew. Levin asked, 'Could you maybe lend us a few slices of bread?'

As usual, I had cooked more than enough. I was just on the point of feigning hospitality when Pavel gave me an admonitory look. I got up to fetch some bread from the larder.

At that, Alma, the model of a charming hostess, said, 'Do sit down. There's plenty here for everybody. Pavel, be a dear and bring another two plates and cutlery.'

Before I could even sit down again, Levin had pulled up two chairs and fetched plates from the cupboard, for Pavel had made no move to get to his feet.

They were starving and in the best of spirits. The usually listless Alma positively blossomed, the children turned silly and fooled around, making a mess of my white tablecloth.

Levin kept casting curious, perhaps even supposed to be wistful, glances around the conservatory. He seemed not to notice my bulge, accepting the presence of the lodgers without the slightest surprise and ignoring Pavel's monosyllabic uncommunicativeness.

Hardly had we swallowed the last mouthful than Pavel leapt to his feet and rather bossily ordered Alma and myself off to bed – we were both in need of an afternoon nap – saying he would clear everything into the kitchen with the assistance of the children. The visitors took the hint of their dismissal.

I left without a word. I had not the slightest desire to get involved in an argument – not with anybody about anything.

'Warm summer sun, shine kindly here . . .' said Pavel as we sat in the garden later, drinking coffee.

Alma, with a glance at my tummy, asked, 'And which of the two young gentlemen is the father?'

Pavel and I exchanged amused looks. 'The lanky one, he's called Levin,' he answered for me.

Alma's interest in the world about her was, thankfully, restricted to this one point; the fact that my husband lived in a separate flat did not seem to have occurred to her. With her tired eyes, she gazed out across the blooming meadow (what once had been Hermann Graber's lawn had been left to run wild) and was apparently enjoying her coffee, the sunshine and her liberty. Her white hand lay limp on Pavel's arm; I preferred not to look at it. And to make matters worse, my inscrutable cat, too, seemed to have taken an interest in her, having ensconced himself snugly on her lap, not purring, but blinking watchfully all around.

Suddenly Lene staggered towards us, sobbing breathlessly, 'It's Kolya!'

Pavel and I leapt to our feet and rushed in the direction of Lene's pointing finger. The llama didn't so much as budge.

Kolya had fallen out of the tree. He had a cut on his head which was bleeding, but didn't seem serious. 'I need a sticking-plaster,' the brave little soldier said.

Pavel carried him into the house, and I snipped off a clump of his hair and pressed a clean kitchen towel on to the wound.

Pavel decided that the gaping cut would need stitches. I put a bandage on it, and he drove off to the hospital with his son.

Lene had cried inconsolably as she watched the patching up going on, so now I took her comfortingly in my arms and went back out to our sunny spot in the garden. I was puzzled at Alma's total lack of interest in Kolya's accident. But she was no longer sitting stoically, as expected, in her basket chair. She had disappeared. I set off at once in search of her, but couldn't find her either in the garden or in the house.

Had Alma slipped into the car beside Pavel?

I sat down on the stairs, brooding. Lene was gradually calming down, and I didn't want to get her worked up again by hunting around feverishly. But then, quite off her own bat, she asked, 'Did Mummy go in the car, too?'

'Yes,' I assured her.

How long would Pavel be away? I knew that at the week-ends there was always a considerable gathering of patients in the accident and emergency waiting-room at the hospital – footballers, amateur gardeners and the odd guilt-stricken father who had accidentally dislocated his little daughter's arm while horsing around with her.

I was bothered about Alma. Once again, taking Lene by the hand, I trailed through the shrubbery, up and down the street, down into the cellar, through all the rooms. We're looking for the cat, I convinced her. In the end, and much against my better instincts, but, desperate for any kind of help, I knocked on Levin's living-room door. The very moment he opened it, I could hear – with boundless relief – a woman's voice. Alma was sitting with the two 'young gentlemen' in front of the television set. 'I just wanted to make sure . . .' I started to say.

'Come and join us,' said Levin. 'We're watching a tennis match.'

I shook my head and left. Once downstairs again, I reproached myself. Levin and his travelling companion knew nothing of Alma's psychosis. So long as they didn't give her anything alcoholic to drink. Hadn't Levin been holding a whisky glass in his hand? Alma was under psychiatric drugs.

An hour and a half later, Pavel returned. Without having to be told, Kolya put on his pyjamas, quite happy to be treated as the wounded hero. He didn't even ask for his mother.

'Alma's upstairs, glued to the television,' I said to Pavel.

Shooting me a look that was far from friendly, he set off up the stairs.

When he brought his wife back down, she was in remarkably high spirits. Without second bidding, Lene told her about Kolya's fall. Strangely enough, his mother burst out in loud laughter at this, while Pavel and I looked at each other in dismay.

'When do we eat?' asked Alma. From her time in hospital, she was accustomed to having the last meal of the day early and going off to bed promptly.

Pavel went into the kitchen, while I laid the table.

'Wrong,' said Alma. 'Two plates too few.'

'Levin and his friend will be eating upstairs,' I said firmly, and tears welled up in her eyes.

Pavel stroked her like some pet animal and passed her three different kinds of pills, which she swallowed obediently. After the meal, she went off peaceably to bed, while we sat on together with the children and listened for the fifth time to the story of Kolya's fall.

When it was bedtime at last, we had to change all the arrangements yet again. I moved into the little study. Alma was already asleep in my double bed when the children slipped in beside her. They had never taken to the attic room, which now fell to Pavel's lot.

I was wakened in the middle of the night. The light was on, and she was standing in front of me. It was like the extension of a dream. Creatures like her are the sort of people who, in stories set in the States of the American Deep South, are usually put to bed by their black slaves – white and apathetic, with flowing hair that has been brushed to a shine by their nanny.

'Where is Pavel?' she asked, staring at the bed as if he had crept under my blanket. For the very first time, I detected mistrust in her features.

'He's in Kolya's bed, up in the attic.'

She sat down on the edge of my bed. 'And where does your husband sleep?'

Drowsily, I pointed upwards; the details were none of Alma's business.

'Queer, is he?' she asked brightly.

I shook my head and shut my eyes, a heavy hint.

She got the message and turned to leave. 'By the way, the young gentlemen are not in the least boring,' was her fatuous parting remark.

As sleep returned, I had the passing thought that 'Désirée' would be a fitting name for her.

We all slept late. As it turned out, the children were the first to get up, and they went outside to play football. This, despite the fact that Kolya had been given strict orders not to do anything strenuous. Still sleepy, I got out of bed, whistled to the children to come inside, and went into the shower, pondering the question of whether I should boil eggs for breakfast.

This time tomorrow, you'll be shot of her, I consoled myself. It was one thing to run about after a man and two children, but a crazy female on top of that? And besides, I found her spoilt and bone idle. She seemed to be exploiting her illness to the very limit, so as to avoid both responsibility and the simplest of tasks, and to be able to lead the pleasurable existence of a pampered child.

Pavel, too, got up and gave me a hand. 'I hope this weekend will be the first and last time she'll be here,' he said. 'We've got to find another solution.'

Like the children, Alma drank cocoa at breakfast. Quite out of the blue, she started bombarding her son, still the worse for wear, with sums, which he solved sullenly at first, before refusing altogether to do any more.

'Leave him be, it's Sunday after all,' said Pavel.

So she went over and lay down in the hammock with Tamerlane, and watched while we cleared the table. I was desperate to go for a walk on my own, but Lene tagged along.

On our return, we found Kolya and Pavel sitting in front of the television, watching a cartoon, and Lene was peeved at having missed half of it. Where was Alma?

'Sleeping.'

Suspicious, I searched the hammock and all my other beds. Obviously, she was upstairs again. I informed Pavel of this.

His brow furrowed darkly. 'Would you go and get her, please, I'm so sick of it all . . .'

So was I, but I did as he asked. I needed neither to knock nor to ring; all the doors were wide open. They didn't notice me, since they were chatting loudly while the radio blared.

'The baby's not mine,' I heard Levin saying.

Roars of laughter all round. Alma chirruped some comment.

'Quite right, it's mine,' said the stranger, and this was apparently just as witty as the old one about the 'paper hashy angel'.

Without their having noticed me, I slipped back downstairs. I went into my bedroom, locked the door and had a good bawl at the depths to which people could sink. Was it supposed to be my problem if the llama was up there drinking beer? Never again would I set foot in Levin's flat of my own accord.

Sooner or later, I don't know when, Pavel was hammering on my door. I opened it. Oh, somewhere on the stairs I had felt a premature contraction, I lied. Pavel became concerned, started blaming himself and his family and went off to fetch Alma.

When we had gathered together again for lunch, she appeared agitated, in a bit of a huff, and her customary lethargy seemed to have fallen from her.

Pavel was watching her with some suspicion. 'Don't you think it would be better if I drove you back today instead of tomorrow?' he asked, his voice soothing. 'It's all rather tiring for you.'

'Are you all trying to get rid of me? A promise is a promise,' she said with surprising self-assurance.

Where I was concerned, she acted with tetchy ill-humour; a reaction to my place in her family, which struck me as much more normal than her previous indifference.

When Alma didn't return from the toilet, but instead seemed to have slipped upstairs again, despite this having been strictly forbidden, Pavel threw in the towel. 'Obviously she likes it up there,' he said. 'I'm fed up with running around after her. And anyway, I'm sure they wouldn't exactly . . .'

I said nothing. The trouble was that Levin had no idea of the kind of person he was dealing with. Without so much as thinking, he would offer her a joint or a whisky. But was *I* supposed to be the one responsible for Alma's welfare?

She spent her days in a women's wing and, apart from doctors and male nurses, seldom set eyes on a man. Besides,

I could hardly believe she would try to make Pavel jealous or to pay him back for any possible unfaithfulness. It was more a case of her behaving like some five-year-old who, never having had any sense of modesty dinned into her, simply enjoys lively male company. And of course it was fun for Levin and his new friend to receive a female visitor, especially because Pavel so obviously disapproved. Just what sort of things could Alma be telling them?

'I doubt very much whether Alma's doctors' plan is going to work,' said Pavel. 'They're trying to ease her way back into everyday life by gradual acclimatization. In fact, the intervals are getting longer, and perhaps it might never come to another severe attack. But when I see her like this, it worries me no end.'

He was right. I, too, had the feeling she couldn't, with an easy conscience, be left on her own for long, nor for that matter alone with the children. And yet she hadn't done anything out of order, nor was her speech confused. In fact, if you disregarded her fixed stare, she was even quite impressive from a distance.

'My God,' said Pavel. 'You should have seen her when we first got married. Everyone envied me my wife: beautiful, intelligent, charming, witty. Sometimes I feel like throwing away these damned pills that have switched off her personality and are making her into a puppet of the pharmaceuticals industry.'

The afternoon went off without a hitch. Alma went for a walk with her family, while I stayed home and rested. The Porsche, too, was gone. Once I had spent a couple of hours just lazing around, I found myself beginning to look forward to my visitors' return.

Although Alma was physically exhausted after the long walk, her increasing restlessness became clearly noticeable. I knew what she would do the next time she had the chance. And sure enough, she soon slipped away out of the living room, only to return almost immediately, looking extremely disappointed.

Now and then I got the feeling she was watching me.

* * *

At this, perhaps not especially exciting, point, I was again rudely interrupted by Rosemarie's loud snores. Cut to the quick, I shut up.

20

At breakfast, Rosemarie was shamefaced. 'It was nothing to do with you, the fact that I fell asleep. I'm sure it's because of that hormone injection.'

She might well have been right, at that. In a way, I felt touched by the way she guiltily tossed her pack of strawberry jam and her sugar lumps on to my bed.

'Tell you what,' I suggested, 'I'll name my daughter after you; not your second name – Thyra is a bit too out of the ordinary for my taste – but half of Rosemarie.'

'Which half?' she asked, delighted.

'She'll be a little Marie.'

'Well, we're going to have to drink to that!' We clattered our thick cups together. A splash of ersatz coffee, livened up with Nescafé, landed on her apricot-coloured sleeve.

'But today we have to get to the end,' she said. 'I take it there are more corpses to come.'

'Wait and see.'

For the evening meal, I served up smoked salmon with a dill sauce.

'The condemned woman's last meal,' said Alma, no doubt thinking ahead to the meagre fare awaiting her in the institution.

Again, she was the first to go to bed, and the children followed. Around midnight, I was wakened by a horrendous dream. I couldn't remember in exact detail, but it began harmlessly enough: Alma and Tamerlane (in human size) were standing there before me, arm in arm, saying, 'We've decided to get married!' Tamerlane was wearing thigh-boots, as befits a cat, as well as the Walt Disney version of a Robin Hood costume. Alma was done up as a deathly pale Snow White. 'Give me Tamerlane to be my husband, and then you can have Pavel,' she was saying, at which I expressed my delight over this fair exchange.

'To make sure it really is fair,' she went on, 'I have taken your child as a bonus.'

I flew into a panic and began desperately searching for my baby in an icy cold forest full of dead trees.

'Just like a fairy story that ends unhappily!' I groaned, trying to wake up. I got up at once, went into the kitchen, drank a glass of milk, looked in on the children – who were sleeping peacefully beside Alma in the double bed – and gazed out of the darkened window.

The Porsche swept into the drive. 'Too late, young gentlemen,' I thought. Finally, I crept into the conservatory. Pavel was lying in the hammock, reading. We snuggled up together. Until Tamerlane, who was able to open doors, stood before us, letting out a tiny sound. I looked up and caught sight of Alma in her lacy nightdress, standing motionless in the empty hall.

Pavel let go of me at once and leapt to his feet. 'What's the matter? Can't you sleep?' he asked awkwardly.

She looked at us as if mortally wounded and disappeared again, as indeed did I, too. Even with my eyes closed, I could still see this desperately unhappy vision before me.

A few hours later – it must have been about three – I was roused again. The cat leapt with a thump on to my chest, which was not his usual way. I stroked his fur. Tamerlane disliked visitors, almost as a matter of principle, and on top of that, my own edginess transmitted itself to him. He wouldn't leave me in peace, but kept nudging me with his nose. I put on the light and looked at the time. Suddenly, I smelt it, and was immediately wide awake.

In the hall, the smoke was much thicker; coughing, I ran into my bedroom. Alma was missing. Roughly, I shook the sleeping children awake. 'Get dressed, quickly,' I ordered as I ran to Pavel, who had fallen asleep in the hammock.

He was alert at once, wrapped the children in blankets, took them out to the car and parked it fifty metres further down the street. By this time, I had called the fire brigade.

A few moments later, I was hammering on Levin's locked door. I could hear the fire raging in the attic, and now it was eating its way down the wooden staircase. Pavel yelled out to Alma.

It took an age before the two men appeared at the door, dressed only in their underpants. Alma wasn't with them. I didn't need to explain what was going on.

Amazingly, Levin remained calm. 'The smoke is bad for you,' he said. 'You've got to get out into the open at once. We'll take care of everything.' First, he drove the Porsche and Dieter's Mercedes out of the driveway, to clear the way for the fire engine. Then he started throwing clothing and shoes out of the window.

The fact that my jewellery, my photo albums and even some books and a few keepsakes were saved, I owe to Levin's travelling companion. With incredible alacrity, he had managed to make exactly the right choices and carried everything outside in a plastic bath and two suitcases even before the fire engines arrived.

The firemen asked whether anyone was missing and then, wearing heavy breathing apparatus, went into the house. The wainscoting, the parquet flooring, the wooden panelled ceilings, the fitted cupboards, the curtains, carpets and beds were blazing on all floors, while the staircase had been transformed into the jaws of hell. Neighbours had gathered out in the street and watched with me as glowing sparks rose from the luridly lit house like soap bubbles, before falling back into the inferno. 'Isn't it lovely?' said Lene.

If Alma had been in the attic, said the firemen who were trying to make their way inside from the huge turntable ladder, there would be little hope of saving her now.

Pavel was in a state of shock.

It was Levin who caught sight of the phosphorescent eyes of the cat, shining in the darkness under the big pine tree. He was about to pick up the terrified animal when he discovered Alma. She had been overcome by the smoke and had burns all over her body, but was still conscious. Pavel held her, motionless, in his arms. The firemen radioed for an ambulance.

'I wanted to kill myself,' said Alma.

She was taken to the hospital in Oggersheim, while I went with Lene to Dorit's and Pavel drove with his son to a colleague of his. Where Levin spent that night, I still don't know to this day. My house was beyond saving, and burned to the ground. In the attic, petrol had been scattered around.

Perhaps I shall get over it in time, and perhaps, too, the memory of all the incidents that took place in that house will fade.

Later on, we heard from Alma herself that, after her appearance in the conservatory that night, she had gone up to see the men, to say her farewells. Together, they had drunk a bottle of Slivovitz. Levin had put it into her head that Pavel was the father of my baby.

With the cash I already had, plus the money from the fire insurance, I subsequently bought a house in the 'Nibelungen' estate in Weinheim, where Pavel and I now live an agreeable, thoroughly middle-class life with Kolya, Lene, Niklas and Tamerlane. Like thousands of other mothers, I open my own mouth wide as I feed my child, cut Kolya's mop of hair (which tends to be shaggy, just like his father's) and lick the blobs of jam off Lene's little hands every morning after breakfast. As far as my doctorate is concerned, I doubt if I'll ever have time for it again. Now and again, I get a postcard from North Germany, where Levin and Dieter run a used-car business. I advanced them the start-up capital for it.

'So just who is little Niklas's father, then?' asks Rosemarie.

'I don't know, and I don't want to know. The only thing that matters is that Pavel is little Marie's father.'

'So that's it?' asks Rosemarie. 'All's well that ends well?'

'Depends on how you look at it. In my parents' eyes, I'm beyond

190

the pale, since both Pavel and I are still married, only not to each other, unfortunately.'

Rosemarie says nothing. Is she really taking it all in? In an hour, a taxi will be coming to take her home. Before that, she wants to have her meal here. So as to economize at home, I suppose.

Our lunch is brought to us, and she peers inquisitively under the serving cover: we're having, as we've already had three times, meatballs with a caper sauce. I push it around my plate; it would need a bit more salt, a bayleaf and a few drops of lemon juice to make it edible.

Rosemarie, who is no cook, has few objections to make about the insipid hospital fare as a rule, but she can't stand capers.

Meticulously, she removes these dark little spheres from the meat and the gravy and sweeps them to the edge of her plate with her fork.

'I suppose everything your grandfather left you went up in smoke too, didn't it?' Obviously she has been paying closer attention than I would have liked.

'The foundations of my villa were still standing. After Niklas was born, healthy and without any complications, I went back one day to scour around in what had once been my cellar and salvaged a few worthless items, among them a certain flower pot.'

'That's marvellous, Hella. So now I can provide my godchild with a legitimate father . . .'

I've never so much as even mentioned godparents. What is she driving at?

'Can you get a divorce from Levin?'

'Well, yes. He's none too delighted at the prospect of a second little cuckoo in his nest. But what good would it do? Pavel has his scruples about leaving poor, sick Alma.'

'It's Alma I'm talking about. Now look, she enjoys the peppery sausage-spread we get here, right?' Deep in thought, she is poking the capers around in the gravy on her plate. 'I might just have a recipe for you: squeeze some meat out of the sausage skin, substitute two peppercorns right at the end of the sausage with poison inside the shells, refill the skin with the meat . . .'

My meatball sticks in my throat.

Undeterred, and warming to her subject, she goes on, 'And then *off we go! For the four children's sake, we'd be best to take a holiday cottage . . .'*

Nauseated, I choke up the meatball and spit it out on to the swivel tray. All of a sudden, I realize that I shall never touch meat again as long as I live.

'It would take Alma some days to finish up the last of the sausage.'